Structured Exercises in

WELLNESS

Promotion

Volume

5

Structured Exercises in

WELLNESS

Promotion

A Handbook for
Trainers, Educators, Group Leaders

Volume

5

Edited by
Nancy Loving Tubesing, EdD
Sandy Stewart Christian, MSW

REPRODUCTION POLICY

Library of Congress Cataloging in Publication Data

Structured exercises in wellness promotion : A handbook for trainers, educators, and
  group leaders / Nancy Loving Tubesing and Sandy Stewart Christian, eds.
  192p. 23cm.
    Summary: A collection of thiry-six exercises for wellness promotion to be used
by trainers and facilitators in group settings.
  ISBN 1-57025-075-8 (v.5 : pbk) : $29.95
  1. Health-Education, problems, exercises, etc 2. Health—education and
problems. I. Title. II. Tubesing, Nancy Loving   III. Christian, Sandy Stewart
  RA440.5.S77   1986, 1990, 1994, 1994, 1995
  613'.2—dc19
83-61074

Printed in the United States of America

10 9 8 7 6 5 4 3 2 1

Published by: 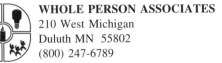 **WHOLE PERSON ASSOCIATES**
210 West Michigan
Duluth MN 55802
(800) 247-6789

PREFACE

Over a decade ago we launched an experiments in education—the Whole Person series of **Structured Exercises in Stress Management** *and* **Structured Exercises in Wellness Promotion.** *We believed that it was time to move beyond peptalks and handouts to an experiential approach that actively involves the participant—as a whole person—in the learning process.*

What began as an experiment has become a catalyst for dramatic change in health promotion and education! **Structured Exercises** *volumes have found their way into the libraries of trainers, consultants, group workers, and health professionals around the world. We're proud that these volumes have become classics—the resource of choice for planning stress management and wellness promotion programs.*

Our purpose in publishing this series was to foster inter-professional networking and to provide a framework though which we can all share our most effective ideas with each other. As you will soon discover, we scoured the country looking for the most innovative, effective teaching designs used by the most creative consultants and trainers in business, health care and social services, then included some of their most imaginative ideas in this volume.

Many of the exercises we designed ourselves and refined in hundreds of workshops we've conducted over the past twenty years. Some are new combinations of time-tested group process activities. Others were submitted by people like you who continually strive to add the creative touch to their teaching.

The layout of **Structured Exercises** *is designed for easy photocopying of worksheets, handouts and preparation notes. Please take advantage of our generous policy for reproduction—but also please be fair to the creative individuals who have so generously shared their ideas with you.*

☞ *You may duplicate worksheets and handouts for use in training or educational events—as long as you use the proper citation as indicated on the copyright page. Please also give written credit to the original contributor. Whenever we've been able to track down the source of an idea, we've noted it. Please do the same when you share these ideas with others.*

☞ *However, all materials in this volume are still protected by copyright. Prior written permission from Whole Person Press is required if you plan large scale reproduction or distribution of any portion of this book. If you wish to include any material or adaptation in another publication, you must have permission in writing before proceeding. Please send us your request and proposal at least thirty days in advance.*

Structured Exercises *are now available in two convenient formats. This small-format softcover version is produced with a new book binding process that says open on your desk or podium for easy reference, and lies flat on the photocopier for quick duplication of worksheets.*

Many trainers enjoy the wide margins and larger type of the full-size looseleaf format, which provides plenty of space for you to add you own workshop designs, examples, chalktalk notes, and process reminders for your presentations. The looseleaf version also includes a complete package of camera-ready worksheet master for easy reproduction of professional looking handouts.

☞ *See page 152 in the Resources section for complete descriptions and ordering information for worksheet masters and companion volumes of the* **Stress** *and* **Wellness** *series in softcover and looseleaf formats.*

We are grateful to the many creative trainers who have go generously shared the "best" with you in this volume (see page 151) as well as others in the series. We hope that the ideas here stimulate your own creative juices.

So go ahead. Strive to bring your teaching alive in new ways. Expand your stress management approach. Continue to touch and motivate people with learning experiences that engage and challenge them as whole persons.

Then let us know what works well for you. We'd love to consider your new ideas for inclusion in a future volume so that we can carry on the tradition of providing this international exchange on innovative teaching designs.

Duluth MN   *Nancy Loving Tubesing*
June 1995   *Sandy Stewart Christian*

INTRODUCTION

Wellness is the hot topic of the decade. If you're prepared to address the issue, you'll get plenty of opportunities. If you creatively involve people in the learning process, reflecting assessing, prioritizing, sorting, planning for change and affirming progress, your teaching will be much more helpful than even the most entertaining lecture.

Structured Exercises in Wellness Promotion, Volume 5 provides 36 designs you can use for getting people involved, whatever the setting and time constraints, whatever the sophistication of the audience. To aid you in the selection of appropriate content and process to meet your objectives, the exercises are grouped into five broad categories:

Icebreakers: These short (10–20 minutes) exercises are designed to introduce people to each other and to open up participants' thinking process regarding wellness. They are lively! Each engages people actively in the topic and with each other. Try combining an icebreaker with an exercise from the wellness or self-care section for an instant evening program.

Wellness Exploration: These exercises explore the issue of wellness from the whole person perspective. Rather than focusing merely on the physical, these processes help people examine their lifestyle. You'll find a mixture of moderate-length assessments (30–60 minutes) and major theme developers (60–90 minutes). Any exercise can easily be contracted or expanded to fit your purpose.

Self-Care Strategies: These exercises promote personal responsibility for well-being. Participants examine their self-care patterns and explore specific self-care strategies in different life dimensions: physical (diet, relaxation, fitness), mental, rational, spiritual and lifestyle well-being. (10–60 minutes)

Action Planning/Closure: These exercises help participants draw together their insights and determine the actions they wish to take on their own behalf. (20–40 minutes)

Energizers: The energizers are designed to perk up the group whenever fatigue sets in. Sprinkle them throughout your program to illustrate skills or concepts. Try one for a change of pace--everyone's juices (including yours!) will be flowing again in 5–10 minutes.

The format is designed for easy use. You'll find that each exercise is described completely, including: goals, group size, time frame, materials needed, step-by-step process instructions and variations.

☞ *Special instructions for the trainer and scripts to be read to the group are typed in italics.*

✔ Questions to ask the group are preceded by a check.

➤ Directions for group activities are indicated by an arrow.

● Mini-lecture notes are preceded by a bullet.

Although the process are primarily described for large groups (25–100 people) workshop setting, most of the exercises work just as well with small groups, and many are appropriate for individual therapy or personal reflection.

If you are teaching the workshop or large group setting, we believe that the use of small discussion groups is the most potent learning structure available to you. We've found that groups of four persons each provide ample air time and a good variety of interaction. If possible, let groups meet together two or three different times during the learning experience before forming new groups.

These personal sharing groups allow people to make positive contact with each other and encourage them to personalize their experience in depth. On evaluation, some people will say, "Drop this," others will say, "Give us more small group time," but most will report that the time you give them to share with each other becomes the heart of the workshop.

If you are working with an intact group of twelve people or less, you may want to keep the whole group together for process and discussion time rather than divide into the suggested four or six person groups.

Each trainer has personal strengths, biases, pet concepts, and processes. We expect and encourage you to expand and modify what you find here to accommodate your style. Adjust the exercises as you see fit. Bring these designs to life for your participants by inserting your own content and examples into your teaching. Experiment!

And when you come up with something new, let us know . . .

CONTENTS

Preface V

Introduction VII

ICEBREAKERS

145 INTRODUCTIONS 9 1

In these three brief get-acquainted processes, participants use the metaphor of a boat to describe their lifestyle (**Anchors Aweigh**), learn each others names and goals (**Imaginary Ball Toss**), and identify a whole person health quality (**I See Myself**). (5–10 minutes)

A Anchors Aweigh 1
B Ball Toss 2
C I See Myself 3

146 FACT OR FICTION 4

In this playful icebreaker, participants answer four questions about their health habits and challenge others to guess which of their responses is untruthful. (10–15 minutes)

147 HEALTH TRANSCRIPT 7

In this unique exercise for getting acquainted, participants pretend they are transfer students at a new school, complete a health transcript, and then discuss their grades in a parent-teacher conference. (15–20 minutes)

148 SELF-ESTEEM PYRAMID 10

Participants build self-esteem by talking about their positive qualities with a growing number of people. (15–20 minutes)

149 TO DO LISTS 12

This simple five question sequence helps people get their priorities in order while they get acquainted. (10–15 minutes)

WELLNESS EXPLORATIONS

150 FAMILY HEALTH TREE 15

Participants discover their family health history by drawing a genogram and recording the medical history of their family over three generations. (50–60 minutes)

151 LIFE THEMES 23

Participants examine positive and negative personal life themes that affect their health and lifestyle, and are challenged to develop more health-promoting themes and new rituals to celebrate them. (90 minutes)

152 PIE CHARTS 33

This adaptable assessment tool uses the symbol of wholeness to explore self-care attitudes and actions. (20–30 minutes)

153 STATE FLAG 37

In this imaginative exercise, participants design a state flag that represents their current state of well-being. (10–15 minutes)

154 WORK APGAR 40

Participants measure their satisfaction with the function of their work systems using a quick, reliable scale, and then explore ways to increase their satisfaction levels on the job. (10–15 minutes)

SELF-CARE STRATEGIES

155 VALUES AND SELF-CARE CHOICES 45

Participants examine what constitutes a value and whether their self-care choices agree with their values. (20–30 minutes)

156 ASSERTIVE CONSUMER 49

This exercise empowers individuals to express their health care needs assertively by writing a letter to people or organizations able to address their concerns. (40–50 minutes)

157 MEALTIME MEDITATION 56

In this relaxing, sensory meditation, participants tune into ways to nurture themselves at mealtime. (10–15 minutes)

158 HEALTHY EXERCISE **61**

This short video and self-analysis process stimulates, inspires, and empowers participants to seek the health benefits of an exercise they can enjoy. (20–60 minutes)

159 IMAGERY FOR A HEALTHY HEART **63**

This directed daydream technique evens out blood pressure and helps maintain open arteries and a strong, healthy heart. (10–15 minutes)

160 SEVENTH INNING STRETCH **68**

In this invigorating exercise, participants combine fantasy with systematic relaxation skills to stretch each muscle group in the body. (5–10 minutes)

161 MENTAL HEALTH INDEX **71**

Participants define mental health, learn about six common mental health problems, assess their own mental health, and discuss strategies for caring for themselves and others when problems occur. (30–45 minutes)

162 SEVEN WAYS OF KNOWING **76**

Participants explore all seven of their intelligences with this creative, affirming tribute to differing gifts. (60–90 minutes)

163 RELATIONSHIP REPORT CARD **85**

Participants examine the health of their primary relationships and friendships by completing a report card covering positive and negative characteristics for each relationship. (30–40 minutes)

164 SPIRITUAL FINGERPRINT **89**

In this playful, right-brain exercise, participants create an art work which symbolizes their current spirituality, and then reflect upon ways to nourish their spirit. (60 minutes)

165 LEISURE PURSUITS **93**

In this expansive assessment and exploration of the needs met by work and play, participants discover their priorities and possibilities for leisure pursuits. (20–30 minutes)

PLANNING/CLOSURE

166 COMMERCIAL SUCCESS 97

This exercise provides a creative way for participants to synthesize learning at the end of a session, working in teams to develop and perform a commercial to sell key ideas to the public. (15–20 minutes)

167 IF . . . THEN 99

This quick and easy planner challenges participants to imagine the consequences of continuing or changing their present health-related behaviors. (15–20 minutes)

168 JUST FOR TODAY 102

This memorable planning process based on the twelve steps challenges participants to make concrete commitments to change. (15–20 minutes)

169 SELF-CARE BOUQUET 106

In this unique process for planning and closure, participants create a metaphorical mixture of flower essences designed to heal their hearts, minds, and spirits. (20–30 minutes)

170 TAKE THE PLEDGE 110

The power of a promise is apparent in this light-hearted closing pledge of allegiance to wellness goals. (10–15 minutes)

GROUP ENERGIZERS

171 CHOOSE WELLNESS ANYWAY 113

This lively exercise engages participants in a high-spirited litany asserting principles of wellness. (5–10 minutes)

172 CLEANSING BREATH 115

Participants experiment with a yoga breathing technique that is a powerful natural tranquilizer. (3–5 minutes)

173 FOR THE HEALTH OF IT 117

Group members are invited to kick up their heels in a dance for fun and fitness. (5–10 minutes)

174 HEALTHY SING-ALONG **119**

Everyone will enjoy this playful song, which is fun to sing and celebrates good health. (3–5 minutes)

175 LUDICROUS WORKSHOPS **121**

In this hilarious exercise, group members create outrageous courses for an absurd continuing education curriculum. (15–20 minutes)

176 NIGHT SKY **124**

In this awe-inspiring guided image, participants search the heavens for a sense of cosmic meaning and connectedness. (8–10 minutes)

177 PERSONAL VITALITY KIT **127**

Everyone receives an envelope of symbolic reminders to stimulate whole person self-care. (5 minutes)

178 SIGHTS FOR SORE EYES **129**

In this revitalizing self-care break, participants practice four techniques for relieving tension and strain in an often-neglected body part. (1–2 minutes each)

179 STIMULATE AND INTEGRATE **132**

This lively exercise provides motion which integrates both sides of the body while stimulating the mind. (4–5 minutes)

180 STRIKE THREE **134**

This touching reading offers a childlike truth about healthy self-esteem. (3 minutes)

RESOURCES

GUIDE TO THE RESOURCE SECTION **135**

TIPS FOR TRAINERS **136**
Engaging All Seven Modes of Intelligence

EDITORS' CHOICE **139**
Four****Exercises: The Best of **Wellness 5**
Especially for the Workplace

WINNING COMBINATIONS **143**

EAP and Health Promotion Presentaiton
Risk Factors and SElf-Care Workshops

ANNOTATED INDEXES **144**

Index to Chalktalks
Index to Demonstrations
Index to Physical Energizers
Index to Mental Energizers
Index to Relaxation Routines

CONTRIBUTORS/EDITORS **151**

WHOLE PERSON PUBLICATIONS **155**

Icebreakers

145 INTRODUCTIONS 9

In these three brief get-acquainted processes, participants use the metaphor of a boat to describe their lifestyle (**Anchors Aweigh**), learn each others names and goals (**Imaginary Ball Toss**), and identify a whole person health quality (**I See Myself**).

GOALS

To get acquainted with other group members.

To warm-up to the subject matter of the session.

GROUP SIZE

Unlimited. **Imaginary Ball Toss** works best with groups of 8–10 participants, but several groups can participate simultaneously.

TIME FRAME

5–10 minutes

MATERIALS NEEDED

I See Myself: Newsprint or blackboard.

Introduction A: ANCHORS AWEIGH

1) The trainer poses a metaphorical question to begin.

    ✔ What type of boat would best describe your lifestyle?

    ☞ *Stimulate ideas for group members, by quickly naming a variety of boats (eg. canoe, speedboat, liferaft, barge, freighter, houseboat, tugboat, sailboat, icebreaker, steamboat, submarine, destroyer, hydroplane, junk, barge, gondola, kayak, oreboat, fishing boat, tanker, yacht, pontoon, life raft, aircraft carrier, etc).*

2) After participants have had a moment to think about their chosen boat, the trainer proceeds with the next instruction.

    ➤ Introduce yourself to the group by stating your name, the type of boat you chose to represent your lifestyle, and a brief explanation of why you picked that particular boat.

    ☞ *In a group larger than 12–15, participants could introduce themselves to the person sitting next to them instead of the entire group.*

VARIATIONS

■ After participants select their boat style, they place themselves in a continuum, along one wall, from slowest to fastest boat. Then they introduce themselves to the person on their left by stating their name, type of boat, a brief explanation of why they chose the boat they did, and why they positioned themselves where they did on the speed continuum.

Introduction B: IMAGINARY BALL TOSS

☞ *Works best with groups of 8–10 people, but several groups can participate simultaneously.*

1) The trainer asks group members to stand in a circle facing each other, and gives directions for the exercise.

➤ Imagine you are holding a ball in your hand.

➤ Introduce yourself to other group members by stating your name and one of your favorite games with a ball, and then throw the imaginary ball to another group member.

➤ Each person should get the ball once and throw it once. Ask if you can't remember who has had the ball.

2) After all group members have had a chance to introduce themselves, the trainer adds another instruction.

➤ Throw the ball to someone and state one thing that you want to get from the workshop.

☞ *Make sure that everyone has the opportunity to throw the ball once.*

VARIATIONS

■ Group members quickly go around the circle, introducing themselves by first name. The last person throws an imaginary ball to one of the group members, stating that person's name out loud. If the person throwing the ball has forgotten a group member's name, or uses the wrong name, the person catching the ball restates their name. That person then throws the ball to someone else, stating that person's name, and so on, until everyone has had a chance to throw the ball. Pick up the pace and continue tossing the ball around very quickly until everyone knows the names of all group members.

Introduction C: I SEE MYSELF

1) The trainer introduces the concepts of body, mind and spirit well-being, inviting participants to brainstorm adjectives that describe "health" in one of the body/mind/spirit categories.

 ☞ *Record all adjectives on newsprint or blackboard, grouping adjectives within the three categories.*

2) The trainer invites participants to choose an adjective to use for introducing themselves.

 ➤ Pick an adjective that applies to you

 ➤ Think of an example from your personal or work life when you exhibited that quality.

 ➤ Introduce yourself to the group, using this format:

   ➣ I see myself as . . .

   ➣ For example, when . . .

VARIATIONS

 ■ Prepare an adjective list in advance and use it as a worksheet. Participants circle the adjectives that apply to them, and then choose one for the introductions in *Step 2*.

*Imaginary Ball Toss was submitted by Krysta Kavenaugh. The process for **I See Myself** is adapted from Lois B. Hart's creative collection, **Connections: 125 Activities for Successful Workshops** (Amherst MA: HRD Press, 1995).*

146 FACT OR FICTION

In this playful icebreaker, participants answer four questions about their health habits and challenge others to guess which of their responses is untruthful.

GOALS

To heighten awareness of health habits and values.

GROUP SIZE

Unlimited.

TIME FRAME

10–15 minutes

MATERIALS NEEDED

One copy of the **Fact or Fiction** worksheet for each participant.

PROCESS

1) The trainer divides the group into teams of four.

   ☞ *Devise a humorous or meaningful way to divide the group. Or just "letter" off (divide total number by 4 and then use that many letters A-B-C-D-E-F-G, etc). Assign a spot in the room for each letter group to gather.*

2) The trainer distributes **Fact or Fiction** worksheets and outlines the purpose of the exercise.

   ● This is an opportunity to share something about yourself with others in your group.

   ● It is also a chance to have some fun as you consider your health habits and patterns.

3) The trainer gives instructions for the reflection worksheet.

   ➤ Read the four questions and consider your answers.

   ➤ In answering the four questions, you must answer three of the questions truthfully and one with a lie—you choose which.

   ➤ Answer each question in writing. Write legibly.

> ➤ Do not discuss your answers with anyone lest you give away your secret untruth.

4) When most people are finished, the trainer gives the next instruction.

➤ Select someone in your group to act as narrator.

➤ Narrators should collect all of your team's worksheets

➤ Focus on one individual at a time, reading all four of their answers while other group members listen and try to guess which of the answers is false.

➤ After everyone has had the opportunity to guess the answer, the group member who completed the worksheet explains which answers are fact, and which answer is fiction.

➤ When the truth has been revealed to the group, the narrator selects the second answer sheet and reads it.

➤ Repeat the process until everyone's facts and fiction has been revealed.

5) The trainer reconvenes the large group for story telling and insight-sharing, asking provocative questions as needed.

✔ What new truths did you learn about members of your group?

✔ What were some of the most outrageous lies you heard in your group?

✔ What was it like to make up a lie about yourself?

6) The trainer concludes by encouraging individuals to respect their curiosity about other group members, and to take the opportunity to get to know more people during the rest of the day.

VARIATIONS

■ Instead of trying to guess which answer to the four questions is false, participants write their answers on a blank sheet of paper, one question at a time. The answers are then drawn out of a hat, and group members try to guess which participant wrote the answer.

This process was adapted from Lyman Coleman.

©1995 Whole Person Press 210 W Michigan Duluth MN 55802   (800) 247-6789

FACT OR FICTION

For breakfast today, I ate . . .	My favorite form of exercise is . . .
The lifestyle habit that keeps me the most healthy is . . .	My hunch is that I will die from . . .

147 HEALTH TRANSCRIPT

In this unique exercise for getting acquainted, participants pretend they are transfer students at a new school, complete a health transcript, and then discuss their grades in a parent-teacher conference.

GOALS

To get acquainted.

To evaluate personal health.

GROUP SIZE

Unlimited.

TIME FRAME

15–20 minutes

MATERIALS NEEDED

One copy of the **Health Transcript** worksheet for each participant.

PROCESS

1) The trainer invites participants to pretend that they are transfer students at a new high school. Their Health Transcript has been sent to the school principal, and will be discussed soon in a parent-teacher conference.

2) The trainer passes out copies of the **Health Transcript** worksheet and explains that in order to prepare for this conference, participants will fill out their own transcripts, and grade themselves in behavior and academic subjects representing whole person health.

   ➤ At the top of the transcript, write your **name**.

   ➤ For the **grading period**, write the time frame that you want to consider for this transcript.

   ➤ You may use this past week, month, year, decade, or your entire life.

   ➤ On the top right corner of your transcript, write the number of days you were **absent** (rebellious) or **tardy** (resistant).

   ➤ Now give yourself a **letter grade** for each academic subject, as well as a grade for extracurricular activities.

   ☞ *Give several examples of behaviors for assessment in each subject area.*

> Give yourself a grade for **achievement, effort, conduct,** and **attitude** for each subject.

> Feel free to add a few comments of explanation, commendation, or exhortation.

3) When everyone has finished, the trainer instructs participants to find someone they do not know well to join them in a parent-teacher conference.

➤ Decide who will be the *Parent*, and who will be the *Teacher*.

➤ The *Teacher* goes first.

> Read your transcript to your *Parent* partner.

> Explain why you chose the grades you did for each subject.

> Share any comments you added.

> Take 5 minutes to describe your transcript.

➤ The *Parent* listens carefully, accepting the *Teacher's* report without criticism or judgement.

> *Parents* may not interrupt *Teachers* except to ask clarifying questions.

➤ When *Teachers* have finished explaining their report cards, *Parents* go next. *Parents* present their own report cards, while *Teachers* listen attentively, without judgement or interruption.

4) After 8–10 minutes, the trainer informs the group that the conference time is up, and invites participants to share general feedback about their conference experiences.

☞ *Acknowledge that some people may not be too happy about their report cards, and encourage them to remember that well-being is an on-going process, not a fixed status. We can always improve our grades in any subject of our health.*

5) The trainer recommends that group members save their report cards, and fill them out again six months from now, to see how their efforts to improve health have paid off.

VARIATIONS

■ Report cards used in an Icebreaker could be saved and then pulled out again for a closing and planning exercise in the same learning experience. Individuals could look over their cards, circle grades or subjects they want to improve, and write behavioral steps for each grading category: achievement, effort, conduct, and attitude.

HEALTH TRANSCRIPT

Name _____

Grading Period _____   Absent _____
                                                        (rebellious)

                                          Tardy _____
                                                        (resistant)

Subject	Achieve-ment	Effort	Conduct	Attitude
General Health *(overall health)*				
Physical Education *(exercise)*				
Home Economics *(nutrition)*				
Chemistry *(chemical use)*				
Sociology *(relationships)*				
Psychology *(mental health)*				
Reading *(intellectual stimulation)*				
Religion *(spiritual values)*				
Art and Music *(creativity)*				
Extracurricular/ Recess *(play)*				

©1995 Whole Person Press 210 W Michigan Duluth MN 55802   (800) 247-6789

148 SELF-ESTEEM PYRAMID

Participants build self-esteem by talking about their positive qualities with a growing number of people.

GOALS

To provide an opportunity for participants to affirm themselves.

To promote group interaction.

GROUP SIZE

Can be adapted to suit most groups.

TIME FRAME

15–20 minutes

PROCESS

1) The trainer instructs participants to pair up with another group member for a get-acquainted affirmation.

 ➤ Each of you has two minutes to say what it is about yourself that you like.

  ➤ You cannot discuss any other topics except yourself—your aspirations, family history, interests, etc.

  ➤ Only positive statements are allowed. No qualifiers, no discounts. No joking.

2) When both individuals have had the opportunity to share their positive qualities, the trainer gives instructions for the second round.

 ➤ Each pair should find another pair and join with them to form a group of four participants.

  ☞ *Encourage people to move quickly. Invite any left out pair to come and join you as a threesome.*

 ➤ Introduce your original partner to the new group, summarizing her positive attributes and strengths.

 ➤ Go around the group until everyone has been introduced.

 ➤ When all introductions are completed, begin a free wheeling discussion about yourselves, emphasizing the qualities that you like about yourself.

☞ *If some groups seem reluctant, encourage them with provocative questions (What skills do you have around the house? At work?), examples, humorous stories, or a role-play demonstration of how the dialogue might sound.*

3) After 5–6 minutes, the trainer interrupts the small group discussions, and instructs each quartet to join up with another foursome to make a group of eight.

☞ *If the numbers don't work out right, create a sextet if necessary.*

4) When everyone has joined an octet, the trainer invites participants to continue their affirmative introductions.

➤ Introduce your original partner to the new group, summarizing her positive qualities and strengths from your original discussion and what you learned about her in the quartet.

➤ Go around the group until everyone has been introduced.

➤ When all introductions are completed, begin a positive, open-ended discussion about yourselves, emphasizing the qualities that you like about yourself.

➤ Do not repeat anything you said earlier.

5) The trainer concludes by pointing out how good it feels to affirm ourselves, and encourages participants to practice this skill throughout the day, noticing how it affects their mood and energy level.

VARIATIONS

■ End the exercise by having participants in the final octets give a sincere compliment to the person sitting on their right. The person who is being complimented has to receive the compliment by listening and then saying "thank you"—and nothing more. No disclaimers allowed!

Submitted by Sandy Queen.

©1995 Whole Person Press 210 W Michigan Duluth MN 55802   (800) 247-6789

149 TO DO LISTS

This simple five question sequence helps people get their priorities in order while they get acquainted.

GOALS

To identify short and long range personal goals.

GROUP SIZE

Unlimited.

TIME FRAME

10–15 minutes

MATERIALS NEEDED

To Do List worksheets.

PROCESS

1) The trainer begins by polling participants on their use of **TO DO** lists.

   ✔ How many of you make TO DO lists? At work? At home?

   ✔ How many of you put "want to" as well as "have to" items on your TO DO lists?

2) The trainer solicits examples of **TO DO** lists and incorporates responses into a brief chalktalk on setting goals and priorities.

   ● If we don't pay attention to goals, they often don't get met. We need to put them on the front burner periodically if we want to make progress.

   ● If our TO DO list is too long, not only do we get discouraged, we also get confused about what to tackle next or waste time fretting about the undone tasks.

   ● Our TO DO lists should include both "want to" opportunities and "have to" obligations. If we don't put healthy recreation or self-nurture activities on the list, we are unlikely to make them a priority.

3) The trainer distributes **TO DO List** worksheets and guides participants through the reflection process.

➤ In the top section, list five tasks that are on your TO DO list for **today**.

   ➢ Your TO DO list might include "want to" playful activities or exciting adventures as well as "have to" unpleasant tasks or dreary obligations.

     ☞ *After this and each of the subsequent questions, pause long enough for nearly all to finish. Remind participants to limit themselves to five—perhaps the five most important.*

➤ In the next section, write down five things TO DO this **week.**

➤ In the next section, identify five things you want TO DO in the **next month**.

➤ In the next section, write down five things you want TO DO **this year**.

➤ In the bottom section, write down five things you want TO DO in your **lifetime**.

4) The trainer invites participants to share some of their TO DO list as a way of getting acquainted in a small group. (5 minutes)

   ☞ *To divide the group, "number" off by days of the week or months of the year (whichever gives you groups of 3–6 people).*

5) The trainer reconvenes the group, asks for examples of goals that might be appropriate to the agenda of the session, then uses these as a springboard to the next content segment.

VARIATIONS

■ The entire exercise could focus on general wellness goals only (eg, five things I want TO DO today/this week/this month/this year/lifetime to improve my health) or a specific area of concern (eg, five things I want TO DO about my fitness, eating patterns, mental health, or stress management, this week/this month/this year/lifetime).

TO DO LIST

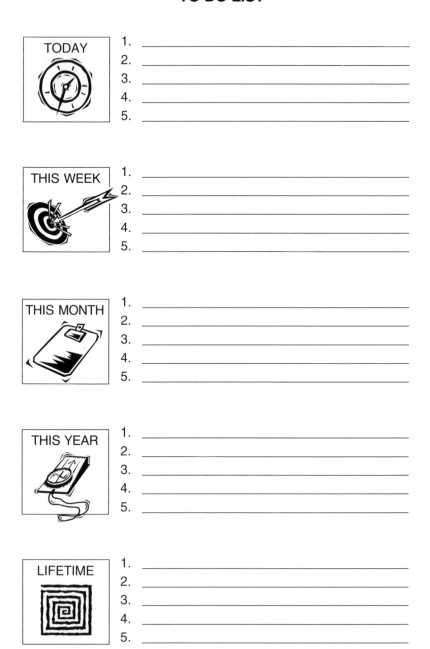

TODAY

1. _____
2. _____
3. _____
4. _____
5. _____

THIS WEEK

1. _____
2. _____
3. _____
4. _____
5. _____

THIS MONTH

1. _____
2. _____
3. _____
4. _____
5. _____

THIS YEAR

1. _____
2. _____
3. _____
4. _____
5. _____

LIFETIME

1. _____
2. _____
3. _____
4. _____
5. _____

Wellness
Exploration

150 FAMILY HEALTH TREE

Participants discover their family health history by drawing a genogram and recording the medical history of their family over three generations.

GOALS

To develop a graphic record of personal medical family history.

To identify any significant health problems or patterns which are present in family health legacies.

To explore possibilities for positive actions which could be taken to reduce inherited health risks.

GROUP SIZE

Unlimited; excellent for individual use.

TIME FRAME

50–60 minutes

MATERIALS NEEDED

One copy of the **Family Health Tree** and **Fruitful Insights** worksheets for each participant.

PROCESS

A. Warm-Up (5–10 minutes)

1) The trainer engages the group by asking participants questions about their health history.

   ✔ How many of you know your cholesterol level?

   ✔ How many of you know your blood pressure?

   ✔ How many of you perform regular self-exams for breast cancer, testicular cancer, or skin cancer?

   ✔ How many of you know the cause of death of your grandparents or great-grandparents?

2) The trainer follows up these questions with a brief chalk talk about health histories and the benefits of knowing about weak and strong links in your family tree.

● **It is not unusual for us to be in the dark about your family health
  history.** Reasons for this may be due to the following:
  Failure to ask (I never thought of it).
  Family secrecy (Don't ask, don't tell).
  Difficulty obtaining medical records (Lost in the war).
  Denial (What I don't know won't hurt me).
  Apathy (Who cares?).
  Assumption that such information is not relevant (It won't affect me).

● **Ignorance is not bliss** when it comes to your health history—it is
  dangerous. A family history of hypertension is a red flag for extra
  precautions in handling stress, controlling weight, exercising regularly. A history of chemical dependency is an obvious clue for
  avoidance of additive substances.

● **We inherit genetic and behavior patterns from our families that
  impact our health.** Heart problems, diabetes, sickle-cell anemia,
  cancer, and many other health problems run in families. Lifestyle
  problems, such as overeating, gambling, and workaholism, are
  inherited by osmosis, as we live with our families and learn from their
  decisions and actions over time.

● **We inherit the good along with the bad.** Longevity, strong immune
  systems, an athletic body, intelligence, and other physical and mental
  attributes also run in families, along with the nurturing of desirable
  qualities like curiosity, a sense of humor, and spiritual faith.

● **Knowing your family health history can empower you to plan** for
  your health and the health of your children. When you know your
  vulnerabilities and strengths, you can make better choices about your
  health and lifestyle. You can seek appropriate medical evaluation, be
  diligent about regular exams, and be intentional about preventative
  measures you can do now.

B. Exploring Your Family Health System (30–35 minutes)

3) The trainer distributes copies of the **Family Health Tree** worksheet to
   each participant, and explains the history and purpose of the genogram,

   ● **A genogram is graphic representation of a family system for over
     at least three generations.** It is a drawing that records information
     about each family member and their legal and biological relationship
     to other members of the family. This format comes out of the work of
     Murray Bowen, psychiatrist, researcher, writer, and pioneer in family
     systems theory.

The genogram was developed to give a quick summary of complex family processes and a source of information about how specific conditions are related to family history and dynamics.

● The genogram can be used to record facts of important life transitions like births and deaths, as well as subjective perceptions you may have about the attitudes and behaviors of family members. As used here, we will focus only on the medical facts.

4) The trainer notes that participants who are adopted should decide whether they want to diagram their adoptive families or their biological families.

☞ *Many adopted individuals do not have access to detailed medical history of their biological parents and grandparents. This frustration could be acknowledged, along with reassurance that they can still glean valuable information by recording their adoptive family's history.*

5) The trainer draws a sample genogram on newsprint and uses it to illustrate how participants can complete their own family trees, beginning with the current generation.

➤ Draw yourself in one of the **My Siblings** boxes at the bottom of your genogram, putting yourself in chronological order of birth, with your oldest sibling on the left and the youngest on the right.

➣ Be sure to include any siblings who died from any cause—including miscarriage and stillbirth.

☞ *Some individuals may be surprised at this last instruction. People may not have thought of deceased children, especially infants or babies who were miscarried, as part of their family. Be prepared to answer questions about why they should be included, with a simple statement explaining that this is an important part of their family medical history.*

For others, there may be a rush of grief if they have not thought about these lost siblings for a long time. In some cases, individuals may never have grieved an infant who died at birth. In addition, there may be family secrets about birth defects or circumstances surrounding the death of a child. Be alert for possible emotional reactions to this portion, and be prepared to offer appropriate support and follow-up for any person in obvious distress.

➣ Use the **square** symbol if you are a male, and the **circle** if you are female, darkening the outline of your gender shape.

(800) 247-6789

☞ *Make sure everyone has done this correctly before moving on.*

➤ Write the first names of your siblings, in birth order, inside the appropriate boxes, and darken their symbol outlines (square for males, circles for females).

➤ If you have more than four siblings, add extra squares or circles as needed for each sibling, in chronological order.

➤ Mark any deceased siblings with an ✗ through their circle or square.

6) When participants have finished their sibling generation diagram, the trainer gives instructions for preceding generation.

➤ Move up to the next generation in the middle of the page, and add your parents, and all of their siblings to your diagram.

➤ Enter the names of all of your aunts and uncles. Mark their gender with circles or squares and put an ✗ in the space of any person who has died.

➤ If you know of miscarriages or stillbirths in your parent's family, draw these in as well.

➤ If you need more boxes, go ahead and add them.

☞ *Advise participants to focus only on their biological or adoptive parents at this level, and to not worry about stepparents unless they can easily add them to the diagram.*

➤ After you have completed drawing your parent's generation, move up to your grandparent's generation at the top of your genogram.

➤ Don't worry about adding the siblings of your grandparents, or the complications of several spouses.

➤ Just record the first names of your grandparents.

7) When participants have finished drawing in all of the people in their family tree, the trainer announces that it is time to add some leaves to the branches of their tree, by filling in the details of their medical history.

➤ Start with yourself by recording the following information beside your symbol on the family tree.

➤ Date of birth.

➤ Significant illnesses you suffered, including dates of onset and your age at the time.

➤ Include emotional or mental illness such as depression, phobias, panic attacks, and other problems.

➤ Note addictions to alcoholism, smoking, compulsive eating, and gambling.

☞ *To help people remember what data to record, post the list where all can see. Be sure everyone is on the right track before moving to the next instruction.*

➤ Record this same medical information (birthdate, physical and mental illnesses with dates, addictions) for every member of your family, working from the bottom of the page to the top, filling in as much as you can remember about these relatives.

➢ For relatives who are deceased, add the date of their death, the age they were at the time of their death, and the cause of their death.

➢ Be sure to record any illnesses that these deceased relatives may have had, and the age they were when they developed symptoms or illness, if you know this information.

☞ *Participants may discover that they are lacking information, and this can be frustrating. Encourage them to do the best they can for now. They can fill in more branches at another time, perhaps by talking with other family members.*

➤ When you have recorded medical information for each family member, go back over your genogram and write in dates of marriages, separations, and divorces for each generation.

➢ If you are unsure of dates, make a guess.

8) When participants have completed their genograms, the trainer distributes **Fruitful Insights** worksheets, and leads participants in further exploration of their health inheritance.

➤ Look over your **Family Health Tree**, and try find connections between your own health problems and those of other family members.

➤ Use the blank space in the center of the apple on your **Fruitful Insights** worksheet to write down all of your insights about the legacy for health and illness that you have inherited from your ancestors.

➤ Record any ideas you have for changing, maintaining, or transforming this legacy.

C. Group Sharing About Family History (10–15 minutes)

9) When individuals have finished recording their insights, the trainer asks participants to form small groups according to the country/region of birth of their grandparents, and discuss their family trees.

➤ Each person has the opportunity to share whatever you choose about your family health tree, and any fruitful insights you have discovered in the process.

➤ Begin with the oldest person in the group, and then go in order of age.

➤ Each person should take about 3–4 minutes to talk about your family.

10) The trainer invites participants to share ideas about how they will apply insights from the session, responding to any concerns or questions, and closing with a few tips on exploring your family health history.

● **Learn your family story.** It is part of "you" whether you acknowledge it or not. If you claim it and understand it, you may discover treasures for enriching your life and health.

● **Respect family members.** Relatives who are reluctant to share information may change their minds if you approach them with respect, explain your reason for wanting to know your history, and commit yourself to protecting and honoring their privacy and dignity.

VARIATIONS

■ Participants who would like to pursue this process further could begin with Carol Krause's step-by-step approach in **How Healthy is Your Family Tree?** (New York: Simon & Schuster, 1995.)

TRAINER'S NOTES

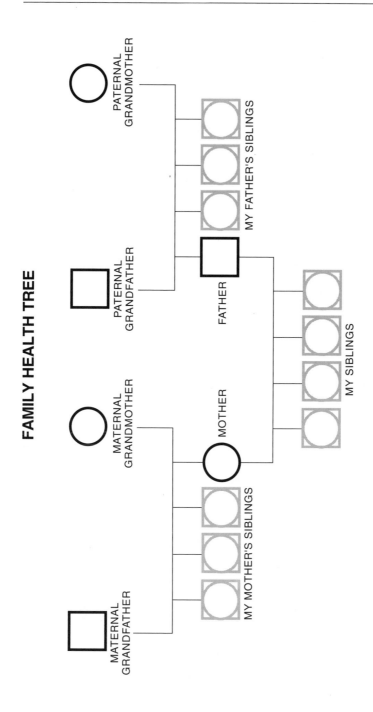

FAMILY HEALTH TREE

PATERNAL GRANDMOTHER

PATERNAL GRANDFATHER

MATERNAL GRANDMOTHER

MATERNAL GRANDFATHER

MY FATHER'S SIBLINGS

FATHER

MOTHER

MY MOTHER'S SIBLINGS

MY SIBLINGS

FRUITFUL INSIGHTS

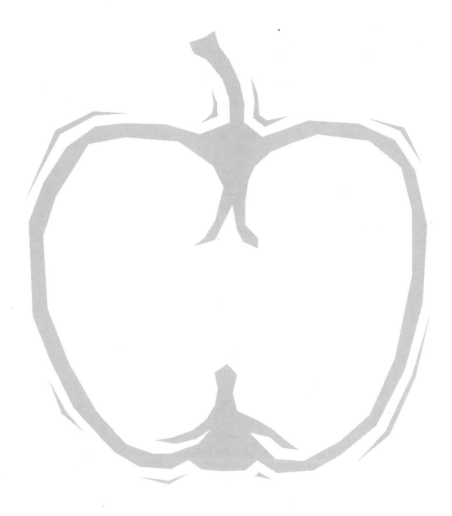

151 LIFE THEMES

Participants examine positive and negative personal life themes that affect their health and lifestyle and are challenged to develop more health-promoting themes and new rituals to celebrate them.

GOALS

To identify negative life themes which may restrict personal growth and health.

To change negative themes to positive, health-promoting themes.

To develop rituals which will enhance healthy life themes.

GROUP SIZE

Unlimited; could be adapted for work with individuals.

TIME FRAME

90 minutes

MATERIALS NEEDED

My Theme Song worksheet and **My Repertoire of Songs and Rituals** worksheet for each participant; newsprint and markers for each small group; blank paper for all participants; a variety of small musical instruments, such as harmonicas, tambourines, bells, horns, etc.

PROCESS

A. Chalktalk and Warm-up to Life Themes (5–10 minutes)

1) The trainer starts with a brief chalktalk about life themes, emphasizing the following points:

● **A theme is like a refrain or chorus that comes back again and again**, in different variations, throughout our lives. Most of us have several life themes learned by osmosis during childhood and played in many variations over the years.

An **abandonment** theme (*I'll die if you leave me!*) might be played out every time you experience a personal loss such as a death, separation from a friend, change of job, or a child leaving home. Instead of viewing these changes as natural life processes, you might instead act out feelings of rejection, hurt, fear, and helplessness.

People with themes of **irresponsibility** (*Eat, drink and be merry!*) might have a long history of failed commitments, unfinished work, and self indulgences, resulting in financial debts, broken relationships, and low self-esteem.

In contrast, a **success theme** (*I can do anything!*) would be marked by a number of achievements that span a person's life history. These folks usually are moving intentionally toward the fulfillment of new goals.

● **Themes are symbolic of underlying attitudes, beliefs, values, and behaviors** which affect our personal health and life style. A person with a **workaholic theme** (*Work 'til you drop*) may have a serious, driven attitude, along with a belief that hard work, success, and achievement are very important. If you live out an **adventure theme** (*Go West, young man!*) you'll probably have optimistic attitudes and a belief that risk-taking and personal challenges are meaningful endeavors. Themes of **giving and caring** for others (*Golden Rule*) may flow out of deep-seated spiritual beliefs.

● **Themes are passed down through the generations**. Consciously or unconsciously, we often carry out these family themes in our current life patterns. Families with themes of **making the world a better place** might raise children who become civic-minded adults, whereas families with themes of **mistrust and self-sufficiency** might produce children who grow into adults with patterns of loneliness and isolation. **Protection** themes might result from a generational avoidance of confronting unacceptable behavior, such as alcohol and drug abuse, by family members.

● **Some themes can be negative or illness-producing**, like a sour note in a song. For example, a theme of **all work and no play** can lead to exhaustion and heart disease. A **denial theme** (*It'll never happen to me!*) can result in ignoring symptoms such as chest pain or a suspicious lump until it's too late.

● **Other themes can be positive and health-enhancing**. These are the sweet notes in the melody of our life patterns. A theme which **celebrates life** could result in many healthy rituals, such as watching the sunrise, spending quality time with family and friends, singing, and praying. An **outdoor** theme might lead to healthy exercise like hiking, swimming, and skiing.

● **We can learn to recognize both sweet and sour notes** in our personal life theme songs, and use this awareness to change these negative themes to positive ones. If people understand that they are living out a **shoot myself in the foot theme**, they can consciously work on a new, both feet on the ground, **stand up for myself theme**. An **I'm a failure! theme** can be changed by setting realistic goals and following through on actions needed to achieve them.

● **Changing these themes requires perceptiveness, planning, and practice.** As human beings, we feel comfortable with our life themes and don't often volunteer to change them until they become excruciatingly painful. But there is hope if you follow the three Ps: perceptiveness, planning and practice. One man who practiced not leaving the room when his wife cried was able to develop an **I'm here for you! theme** in his marriage.

B. Reflection and Small Group Brainstorming (15 minutes)

2) The trainer hands out blank sheets of paper to each participant and invites group members to reflect on the themes implicit in their morning activities.

➤ Close your eyes and recall what your morning was like today.

➢ Think about the moment that your woke up, and about all that has happened to you from that moment until now.

☞ *People may need examples to help them get started. Did their family dog chew up their favorite shoe? Did anyone oversleep?*

➤ Open your eyes now and consider your morning from an outsider's viewpoint.

➢ If your morning were a short story, play, or song, what would the theme be?

➢ Jot down your ideas on paper.

☞ *Give examples: themes of Chaos and crisis; Hurry, hurry, hurry; Go for the gusto.*

The purpose here is to create an atmosphere in the group that allows participants to take risks, be playful, open-minded, and respectful. Be sure to mention that there is no right or wrong theme, and that nobody will be judged on their themes. The idea is to explore ideas and share experiences.

3) After 1–2 minutes, the trainer interrupts the personal reflections and asks if anyone wants to share morning themes. The trainer volunteers an example from her own morning to demonstrate.

4) The trainer divides the group into teams of 4–6 participants, passes out newsprint and markers to each group, and guides people in further exploration of health and illness-producing themes.

➤ Introduce yourself by first name and your morning theme.

  ➢ If you didn't think of a theme yet, just make one up now.

  ➢ Go around the group quickly, so you can finish introductions in 1 minute.

➤ When everyone has introduced themselves, decide which person has the funniest morning theme, and appoint this person to be the group recorder. The recorder will take notes on all the group's ideas, and later will report back to the large group on these ideas.

➤ Brainstorm a list of themes which could **restrict your growth** or health. List as many potentially destructive or illness-producing theme ideas as you can, without censoring or judging them.

  ➢ Take 4 minutes to make your list.

➤ The recorder should list all group ideas on newsprint.

  ☞ *Give some examples to stimulate thinking, using themes which are suited to the audience. For example, a corporate setting might identify with themes such as Do more, Show your worth, Onward and upward.*

5) After about 5 minutes the trainer interrupts with the next assignment.

➤ Look over your list and select the **three most destructive** or illness-producing themes.

6) When groups have made their selections, the trainer invites group reporters to report to the large group on their **top three negative theme**s. The trainer writes these themes on a large newsprint and highlights common group themes as they are revealed in the process.

➤ Now brainstorm a list of life themes which you consider **healthy** and **growth-enhancing**.

➤ List as many ideas as possible in 4 minutes. The recorder should write down all themes on newsprint.

  ☞ *Again, prompt with a few examples appropriate for your audience: Balance, Diversity or Commitment themes.*

➤ Take another 2 minutes to select your **top three health-promoting themes**.

7) When groups have made their selections the trainer invites each group to share their **top three healthy themes,** lists them on newsprint beside

the negative themes, compares the two lists and points out the difference between illness and health themes.

☞ *It is important to state that what is health-promoting for one individual may be illness-producing for another and affirm the right of participants to decide what they consider healthy or unhealthy themes.*

C. My Life Theme Songs Worksheet (25 minutes)

8) The trainer distributes the **My Theme Song** worksheets and guides participants through the reflection process.

➤ Reflect on the history of your path of health and wellness. Recall times when you struggled with health issues and concerns.

➤ Select an incident or dilemma which stands out for you.

 ➣ It may be a time when you faced a serious illness, or a difficult choice about your lifestyle.

 ➣ It could be a time that you felt challenged about your health patterns or choices.

  ☞ *Remind people that this can be a physical, emotional, relational mental or spiritual health issue. Give examples, such as a spiritual crisis when they lost their purpose or meaning, or a mental health crisis, when they became depressed or anxious.*

➤ Write a short story about this dilemma or crisis. Try to include a beginning, middle, and end to the story.

 ➣ Write quickly, without thinking too hard or censoring your thoughts.

 ➣ You will not be graded or judged on your literary skills. A rough outline form or notes are fine. The goal is to recall enough details to develop the story for yourself.

  ☞ *Allow about 5 minutes for group members to write their stories. Remind people of the time when they have about one minute left.*

➤ Look over the list of themes on the bottom half of your page.

 ➣ Circle any which you think are reflected in the theme song story that you have just written.

 ➣ Put a star beside the ones which are major themes for you.

 ➣ Put a check mark beside the ones which are minor themes for you.

©1995 Whole Person Press 210 W Michigan Duluth MN 55802   (800) 247-6789

➤ If you think of any personal life themes which are not listed on the page, add them to the list and mark them with a star or circle.

9) The trainer distributes the **My Repertoire of Songs and Rituals** worksheet and gives instructions for completing it.

➤ Using your **Theme Song** worksheet as a reference, write down your **major** and **minor life themes** in the designated boxes.

➤ Look over your major and minor themes. Are they positive and health-enhancing or negative and illness-producing?

➤ Put a plus sign by the positive, health promoting themes of your life.

➤ Circle the themes you think are negative or harmful to your health.

10) The trainer defines rituals in a chalktalk, using the following points:

● Our themes—major and minor, positive and negative—are acted out symbolically through rituals. **Success themes** may be symbolized by rituals such as graduation ceremonies, awards, blue ribbons, promotions, words of praise, and other special recognitions. **Abandonment themes** might be played out by rituals of crying, sleepless nights, pacing the floor, nail-biting, and eating.

● **A ritual is an action, ceremony, or custom** which is used to mark important events, changes, beliefs, and relationship patterns in our lives. **Loving themes** might include rituals of daily hugs, weekly dates, or special couple events such as a Sunday morning brunch, and backrubs. A family with a **stick together them**e would have many rituals to celebrate transitions in the lives of family members, such as celebrating birthdays together, sharing holiday meals, reunions, and family gatherings during times of crisis..

● **Rituals are often habits that we repeat over and over**, in response to various life themes. If a person's life theme is *Big girls don't cry*, an accompanying ritual might be swallowing tears, leaving the room, and seeking a diversion from emotions, cleaning, joking, or other distractions from pain. A personal life theme of **hospitality** might lead to social rituals of entertaining, visiting new neighbors, and volunteer activities

● **Like themes, rituals can also be illness-producing or health-promoting.** A life theme of **I'm in charge here** might lead to rituals of controlling, bullying, put downs, and even physical violence. Individuals with **playful life theme**s could have healthy rituals of playing on a church softball league, Friday night country dancing , summer camping trips, and weekly massages. A playful life theme could also have unhealthy rituals of excessive drinking after sporting events, partying all night several nights a week, and overspending on recreational vehicles or other toys.

➤ Use the second column to write a few examples of rituals which you usually associate with each of your major and minor life themes.

☞ *Give more examples to stimulate ideas: shopping sprees, watching home movies, baking, etc.*

● **By consciously changing negative rituals to positive ones, we can add healthy notes to our theme songs**, and create music that gives us satisfaction, meaning, and reinforcement for healthy themes. Attending a support group could become a ritual which interrupts a **loneliness** theme. Developing a negotiation ritual for resolving conflicts could interrupt the win or lose dynamics of a **competitive** life theme. Daily walks to replace snacking rituals would enhance healthy themes of fitness.

➤ For each of your major and minor life themes, dream up a new, healthy ritual you could use to celebrate that theme.

➤ Record your ideas in the third column of the worksheet.

➤ Be creative! Imagine outrageous rituals, and have fun with this part. Shake loose from old ways, and develop new methods to enhance your healthy themes and transform your unhealthy themes.

D. New Theme Songs for Health (25–40 minutes)

11) The trainer invites people to stand up, take a quick stretch, and then rejoin their small group for sharing and creative activity.

➤ Allow each person in the group two minutes to share whatever they want about their themes and rituals.

☞ *Monitor the time and encourage groups to stay up with the pace. When most have finished sharing, outline the next step.*

➤ Create a short, one-minute health promoting theme song for your group. You have 10 minutes to create your health song, and then perform it for the large group.

➤ Use a simple melody that everyone knows and try to incorporate some of your group's healthy themes and ritual ideas.

➤ Use musical aids if desired, and symbolic actions to choreograph your song.

12) The trainer invites each group to sing their song for the large group, encouraging raucous applause for each performance.

13) The trainer thanks participants for their creativity in writing and singing songs for health, and concludes the session with a chalktalk suggesting that they use the three Ps—perceptiveness, planning, and practice—to develop healthy themes for their lives.

● **Perceptiveness**. Pay attention to your personal life themes and rituals. Ask yourself if these themes and rituals work for you and provide a healthy, satisfying lifestyle.

● **Planning**. Be intentional. Abandon unhealthy life themes if necessary, even if you inherited them from your family. Choose new life themes that will enhance your remaining years. Reduce the frequency of unhealthy rituals. Replace them with rituals you know will enhance your health and well-being.

● **Practice**. Practice. Practice. Practice until new life themes fit comfortably and your repertoire of rituals offers tons of exciting and creative, health-enhancing options for celebrating life.

TRAINER'S NOTES

This process was inspired by a workshop given at the 1990 AAMFT convention by Evan Imber-Black, PhD.

MY THEME SONG

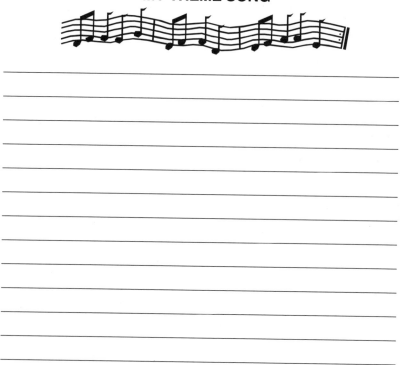

Hero	Nothing can hurt me	Everyone counts—even me
Hospitality	No tears allowed	Small acts don't count
Savior	Go easy on yourself	If at first you don't succeed, try, try again
Others first	Whine, whine, whine	When the going gets tough, the tough get going
Patience	I can't stand it	See no evil, speak no evil, hear no evil
Take action	Be in control	Nobody knows the trouble I've seen
Do or die	Be the best	No pain, no gain
Reach out	Cure me, doctor	Big girls and boys don't cry
Plan ahead	Be responsible	I can't do anything right
Have faith	Zippity-do-dah	Somebody is to blame
Love a lot	Suffer in silence	No time—hurry, hurry
Take time	It's my cross to bear	Murphy was right
Do it right	It's a jungle out there	It's my party and I'll cry if I want to
Take risks	Life's a challenge	Laugh and the world laughs with you
Be careful	Nobody loves me	Beggers can't be choosers
Alone again	I think I can	Whistle while you work
Never give up	Put up or shut up	God don't make no junk
Today matters	Go for the gusto	People who need people are the luckiest people
Control yourself	Family loyalty	in the world

©1995 Whole Person Press 210 W Michigan Duluth MN 55802   (800) 247-6789

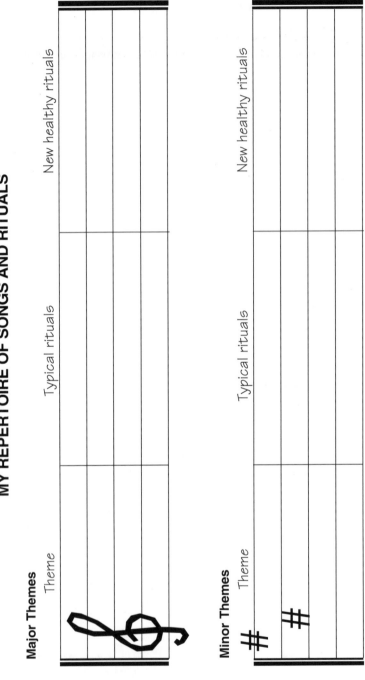

152 PIE CHARTS

This adaptable assessment tool uses the symbol of wholeness to explore self-care attitudes and actions.

GOALS

To explore self-care patterns.

To get acquainted.

TIME FRAME

20–30 minutes

MATERIALS NEEDED

Pie Charts worksheets (duplicated on both sides), chalkboard or newsprint.

PROCESS

☞ *Tailor this generic process to the specific audience, content, and goals you are working with. Be creative in your choice of a second pie chart in Step 6. The suggestions in the Variations are intended to stimulate, not limit your options.*

1) The trainer distributes **Pie Charts** worksheets to all and invites participants to consider the whole of their well-being and their style of whole person health self-care.

● **Health is a whole person issue**. For today, we will be looking at our self-care attitude and actions in six divisions of well-being:
  ○ **Physical health** (fitness, nutrition, disease prevention, relaxation, activity, flexibility, resistance, endurance)
  ○ **Intellectual health** (creativity, problem-solving, eagerness to learn)
  ○ **Emotional health** (managing moods and feelings, personal perspective, capacity to feel deeply, resiliency)
  ○ **Interpersonal health** (nurturing family connections, parenting, capacity to give and receive love, friendship patterns, community)
  ○ **Spiritual health** (ritual, celebration, faith, values, compassion)
  ○ **Lifestyle health** (stress management, work issues, finances, environmental concerns)

    ☞ *Outline these six components and their self-care activities on newsprint or chalkboard for reference.*

● **Each of us has a different agenda for self-care.** Our family heritage and circumstances may dictate how much energy and effort we need to lavish on the various dimensions. Our gifts and capabilities are different as well, so no two individuals will have the same pattern.

2) The trainer give instructions for completing the self-care pie.

➤ Imagine that this circle represents the entire sum of your attention to self-care. From the whole person perspective, include physical, intellectual, emotional, mental and spiritual well-being.

➣ Think about all of your self-care actions—the reading you've done, the courses you've taken, the advice you've sought from professional and nonprofessional sources, the worrying you've done, and the actions you've taken.

➤ Divide your pie into six segments, one for each dimension of self-care. Make the sections proportional to the relative time/energy/attention you give to the six dimensions of self-care.

➣ The light guidelines divide the circle into twelve segments to help you decide proportions.

➣ Draw dark dividing lines that represent the pieces of your pie.

➤ Label each section appropriately with the self-care area name or symbol, then list several examples of your self-care activities in each pie piece.

☞ *Allow 2–4 minutes for participants to complete this task. Encourage people who finish early to go back and add additional self-care examples.*

➤ Now step back and look at your pie. What observations can you make? Write a one sentence analysis of your self-care pie.

3) When nearly all have finished their worksheets, the trainer asks people to stand up and find two partners, making triads.

➤ What's your favorite kind of pie?

➣ With this in mind, find two other people who share your pie passion.

☞ *People may need to choose second-favorite pie fillings in order to find two companions. Do not allow groups larger than three at this stage. A few pairs will work fine.*

➤ As soon as you have a trio, find chairs together and introduce yourselves.

4) As soon as all are settled, the trainer outlines the process for sharing.

➤ Decide quickly who in your group will be ***pumpkin***, ***rhubarb***, and ***lemon meringue***.

> *Pumpkins* will start showing their self-care pie, reading their one sentence, analysis, and elaborating with whatever details you want to share during 2 minutes.

> *Lemon meringues* and *rhubarbs* should listen respectfully and ask clarifying questions along the way, keeping the focus on *pumpkin's* pie.

> After about 2 minutes, I'll give the signal for you to switch roles.

> ☞ *Give a fifteen second warning, then at 2 minutes announce that* ***rhubarbs*** *will share next. Keep time again and announce the third round of sharing after 2 minutes.*

> Now write a second sentence about your pie chart, incorporating any insights you gained while sharing or listening to others.

5) The trainer directs each triad to pair up with a neighboring trio to make a group of six. Participants introduce themselves by reading their second insight sentences.

6) After 2–3 minutes the trainer interrupts and invites participants to create another pie chart, tailored to the specific content of the session.

> ☞ *Ask participants to turn their worksheets over and draw a second pie chart. Give whatever content introduction you want, then repeat the instructions for* ***Step 2*** *and* ***Step 4****, adjusting the directions as necessary to correspond with the new pie. Individuals stay in their sextets for sharing.*

7) The trainer reconvenes group, asks for appropriate insights and responses, weaving them into a bridge to the next agenda item.

VARIATIONS

■ Pie charts are extremely powerful and are infinitely flexible insight generators. Choose one of these for *Step 7* or offer several options for participants to make their own choice.

> *Relationships*: Time and energy spent on your many different relationships (couple friends, extended family, work, church, etc).
> *Food*: Ratio of healthy to junk food.
> *Time expenditure*: In whatever categories make sense.
> *Activity analysis*: Sedentary vs active times (couch potato, moderate slug, busy beaver, etc).
> *Balance*: Investment in work, home, self.
> *Worries*: Groups of issues trigger anxiety.
> *Feelings*: Percentage of time you spend feeling angry, sad, joyful, scared, etc.

PIE CHARTS WORKSHEET

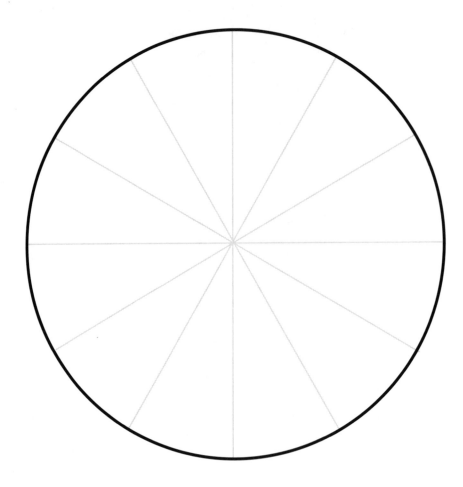

153 STATE FLAG

In this imaginative exercise, participants design a state flag that represents their current state of well-being.

GOALS

To create a visual metaphor for personal wellness.

To provide a playful, nonthreatening way for group members to get acquainted.

GROUP SIZE

Unlimited.

TIME FRAME

10–15 minutes

MATERIALS NEEDED

State of Well-Being Flag worksheet and crayons or colored markers for each participant; reference books (almanac, encyclopedia) with pictures of state flags; masking tape (for **Variation**).

PROCESS

1) The trainer introduces the topic by observing that wellness is an ongoing process that changes from month to month or year to year. She explains that in this exercise, participants will create a metaphor to represent their current state of well-being.

2) She distributes **State of Well-Being Flag** worksheets, and crayons or colored markers to participants, and explains the process.

> Design a state flag that represents your current state of well-being.

> Create a symbol or state seal which reflects your current wellness.

> Write a motto about your health or wellness on your flag.

> Write your name on your flag.

> Include the date that you achieved this state of wellness.

3) The trainer passes around reference books with pictures of flags so people can see some examples of designs and symbols.

4) When participants have finished designing their flags, the trainer gives instructions for forming small groups and sharing.

> ➤ Find three people who were born in the same state as you were (or in a neighboring state).

> ➤ As soon as you have a quartet together, find a spot to sit down and describe your flags to each other.

>> ➣ Each person should take 2 minutes to show your flag and describe your current state of well-being.

>> ➣ Start with the youngest person in your group and take turns by increasing age.

5) The trainer reconvenes the large group and creates a **State of Well-Being** flag for the group, incorporating examples and suggestions from participants.

6) The trainer winds up with a reminder that because wellness is a dynamic, ever-changing process, participants can decide how they would like their state flag to look in six months or a year from now.

VARIATIONS

■ Keep the state flag metaphor but change what it represents. Consider your state of mental health, spiritual health, physical health, relationship health, self-esteem, stress, mind, family health, independence, autonomy, self-hood, identity, self-acceptance, hope, denial, courage, tolerance, interest, curiosity, wonder, self-worth, and order.

■ After *Step 4,* all participants post their flags on the wall and spend the next break time checking out the state of well-being of the entire group.

■ In small groups (fewer than 20 participants), keep everyone together for *Step 4.*

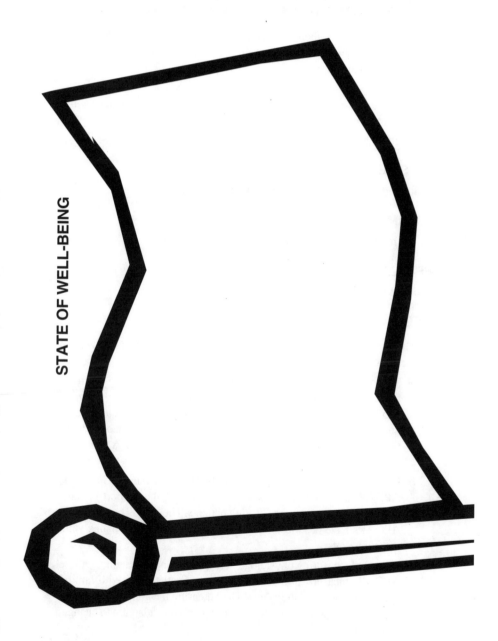

STATE OF WELL-BEING

154 WORK APGAR

Participants measure their satisfaction with the function of their work systems using a quick, reliable scale, and then explore ways to increase their satisfaction levels on the job.

GOALS

To explore satisfaction at work.

To promote healthy work relationships.

GROUP SIZE

Unlimited; also effective with individuals.

TIME FRAME

10–15 minutes

MATERIALS NEEDED

Work APGAR worksheet.

PROCESS

1) The trainer describes the history and purpose of the **Work APGAR** in a brief chalktalk.

   ● The health of a newborn baby is assessed at birth using a simple sequence of observations that is call the APGAR scale. Developed in 1952 by Dr. Virginia Apgar, an anesthesiologist, this unique method quickly rates newborns on five dimensions: **A**ppearance, **P**ulse, **G**rimace, **A**ctivity, and **R**espiratory effect (A-P-G-A-R). A total score of ten is considered topnotch health.

   ● In 1978, family physician Dr. Gabriel Smiklstein, adapted the APGAR model into a quick tool for assessing the support systems (family, friends, and work) of adult patients. These adult psychosocial APGARs have been tested clinically and found to be reliable, valid measurements.

   ● Instead of measuring physiological responses and appearances, these APGARs measure an individual's level of satisfaction with family, friends and work relationships. They measure the ability of a system to provide support, nurturence, problem-solving, adaption to change, and intimacy.

● The **Work APGAR** is a tool that can be used for a quick and easy checkup on your satisfaction with your current work system. There are seven aspects of work which you can evaluate. Your perceptions about how well the system functions will form the basis for your final score.

2) The trainer distributes copies of the **Work APGAR** worksheet, and gives instructions for completing them.

➤ These statements have been designed to help you better understand your work situation.

➤ Answer each of the seven statements about yourself and your work environment.

➣ Check the box which best describes how often you experience satisfaction in the area described by each statement: **most** of the time, **some** of the time, or **all** of the time.

➣ Use the **comment** section if you wish to give additional information or if you wish to describe the way a particular question applies to your work situation.

➣ If you are not currently employed, consider using a work system where you spend time as a volunteer. Or evaluate a system where you have been previously employed.

3) When group members have completed the **Work APGAR** forms, the trainer explains how to score them.

➤ Give yourself:

➣ 2 points for each item that you answered, satisfied **most of the time.**

➣ 1 point for each **some of the time** satisfied answer.

➣ Zero points for each **hardly ever** satisfied answer.

➤ The highest score you could have is 14.

➣ Scores of 0–4 suggest that you are extremely dissatisfied with your work system.

➣ Scores of 5–9 reflect some areas of satisfaction but also some troubling areas.

➣ Scores of 10–14 show a high level of satisfaction with your work system.

☞ *Remind participants that their APGAR scores are a reflection of their current level of satisfaction with their work systems. A low score does not mean that they have done anything wrong. High or low scores can quickly change, depending on a variety of circumstances.*

4) After everyone has scored their **Work APGAR** forms, the trainer instructs participants to divide into 3 groups, based on high (10–14), medium (5–9), and low (0–4) satisfaction scores.

> ☞ *If groups are larger than 6–8 people, divide each level as need to get groups that size.*

➤ Each person has 2 minutes to share your **Work APGAR** scores, along with your thoughts about why you are or are not satisfied with your current work system.

> ➣ Avoid making this a gripe session. Try to describe the circumstances causing your current score without blaming others.

5) When most groups are about finished, the trainer interrupts and invites participants to consider desirable changes.

➤ Select one of the items on the APGAR scale that you were the least satisfied with, and talk about your ideas for raising your level of satisfaction with this score.

➤ If all your scores were high, talk about what you can do to maintain this high level of satisfaction.

➤ Each person has 2 minutes to share your ideas.

6) The trainer invites participants to share ideas for improving their APGAR scores, reminding group members to also consider possible consequences of actions such as confronting a co-worker or supervisor.

7) The trainer concludes with a brief chalktalk, offering encouragement for participants to continue to explore this important area of wellness.

● **Your worksite wellness is important.** Employees who report high levels of satisfaction with their work perform better, have fewer sick days, and are generally less stressed. This spills over into all areas of your life.

● **The health of any system depends upon the health of individuals within it.** Health and wellness are contagious. Make your health a priority, and it is bound to create ripple effects in your work system.

● **Small changes make a difference.** A noontime jog, lunch with a co-worker, or a heart-to-heart talk with a supervisor can improve your satisfaction with your job as much as larger changes or reorganization.

VARIATIONS

■ Work APGAR can be changed into a Family or Friendship APGAR, by using only the first 5 items and replacing the words *fellow workers* with *family* or *friend*.

The scoring method would remain the same, but the highest score would be 10 instead of 14. Scores of 0–3 would be low satisfaction, 4-6 would be a moderate satisfaction, and 7–10 would be a high level of satisfaction.

TRAINER'S NOTES

The Work APGAR and modifications suggested here were developed by Gabriel Smilkstein, Clark Ashworth, and Don Montano.

WORK APGAR

	Most of the time	Some of the time	Hardly ever
1. I am satisfied that I can turn to a fellow worker for help when something is troubling me.	☐	☐	☐
Comments:			
2. I am satisfied with the way my fellow workers talk over things with me and share problems with me.	☐	☐	☐
Comments:			
3. I am satisfied that my fellow workers accept and support my new ideas or thoughts.	☐	☐	☐
Comments:			
4. I am satisfied with the way my fellow workers respond to my emotions, such as anger, sorrow or laughter.	☐	☐	☐
Comments:			
5. I am satisfied with the way my fellow workers and I share time together.	☐	☐	☐
Comments:			
6. I am satisfied with the way I get along with the person who is my closest or immediate supervisor.	☐	☐	☐
Comments:			
7. I am satisfied with the work I do at my place of employment.	☐	☐	☐
Comments:			

The Work APGAR and modifications suggested here were developed by Gabriel Smilkstein, MD, Clark Ashworth, MD, and Don Montano, MD.

Self-Care
Strategies

155 VALUES AND SELF-CARE

In this exercise participants examine what constitutes a value and whether their self-care choices agree with their values.

GOALS

To examine personal values and how they are translated into life choices.

To realign values and act on them.

GROUP SIZE

Unlimited.

TIME FRAME

20–30 minutes

MATERIALS NEEDED

Values and Self-Care Choices worksheets.

PROCESS

1) The trainer introduces the concept of values and self-care choices, emphasizing the following points:

   ● **Values shape our decisions and choices**. Most of the choices we make are based in some way on a belief or value.

   ● Sometimes we are not aware of what our values really are and how they affect our choices. Other times, we may make a choice based on what we think are "good reasons," but that do not agree with our values.

   ● When we feel uncomfortable or unhappy about choices, often it is because of competing or unclear values. What we say we value may not be what we really value. Our actions may be ruled by "shoulds" instead of by what we really believe.

2) The trainer distributes **Values and Self-Care Choices** worksheets and invites participants to consider their self-care priorities.

   ➤ Read over this list of value-related self-care choices.

   ➢ In the empty boxes (E, M, and X), add other self-care values that are important to you.

➤ Now rank the 24 items according to their value or importance to you.

   ➤ In the **upper right corner** of each box, write a number showing how you would rank that value or choice relative to the others on this page.

   ➤ Use 1 as your top priority and 24 as your bottom priority.

➤ Values are more than just saying you believe in something. Consider now your **attitude** about these self-care priorities.

   ➤ Of all the values on the worksheet, find the ones that you endorse joyfully and positively (not the ones you feel you "should" practice).

   ➤ Put a star in these boxes.

3) The trainer divides the groups into pairs and instructs participants to discuss their value rankings, taking into account the following points:

➤ Are the values you marked with stars the same values that you ranked at the top of the list? If not, why not?

➤ Compare your top three choices with your partner's top three. Also compare the bottom three for each. What do you think your choices say about you?

4) After 3–4 minutes the trainer interrupts and notes that the true test of values is whether we **act on them**. Participants are instructed to turn to their worksheets again.

➤ For each value, mark beside its letter label how regularly you act on that self care choice.

   ➤ Use an R for REGULARLY practice it, an S for SOMETIMES practice it, or an N for NEVER practice it.

5) When the action assessment is complete, the trainer asks pairs to join into groups of four and instructs them to discuss their values.

➤ What self-care values did you rank as **unimportant**, even though you regularly practice them? What are the reasons for practicing a value that is not particularly important to you?

➤ What self-care values are ranked high or marked with a star, yet are seldom or never practiced? What are the reasons for that?

➤ What insights have you gained about your values and self-care choices?

6) After 8–10 minutes the trainer reconvenes the large group and directs participants to focus on desired changes.

➤ By now, you may see that you are not acting on some of your important values.

> What single change could you make that is consistent with your highest-ranking values and that would increase your well-being the most?

> Circle that choice on the worksheet.

> At the bottom of the worksheet, write a statement describing the value and telling how you will put the value into action.

☞ *Give an appropriate example. (Eg, "Spirituality is very important to me, so once a day, I will take fifteen minutes for meditation and reflection on the spiritual side of my life.")*

➤ Some changes that reflect lesser-ranking values may still increase your well-being.

> What single change, reflecting one of the values on this worksheet, would be easiest and most efficient to make?

> At the bottom of the worksheet, write a statement describing that value and telling how you will put the value into action.

☞ *Give an example. (Eg, "Wearing a seat belt is not my most important value, but it is an easy choice to make, so I will use my seat belt every time I ride in a car.")*

7) The trainer asks for examples of possible actions from *Step 6*, and concludes with a few summary comments on values and self-care choices.

● Actions that reflect our deeply-held values are easier to sustain than actions that go against our values.

● A value is something that is chosen freely, that makes us feel positive and joyful, and that we practice in our lives. If your values do not meet these three criteria, ask yourself why.

● When we act against our values, we feel "disconnected" and uncomfortable. It may even cause physical symptoms.

● Not all "good" actions have to reflect our most deeply-held values. If a change is positive, easy to make, and doesn't go against your values, why not make the change?

VALUES AND SELF-CARE CHOICES

A Eating a well-balanced diet	B Engaging in spiritual reflection and growth	C Taking responsibility for my own well-being
D Rarely missing work due to sickness	E	F Maintaining an appropriate weight for my height
G Abstaining or using alcohol in moderation	H Engaging in meaningful life work that makes a contribution	I Working to keep my environment free from unnecessary hazards or pollutants
J Regular self-examination for early warning signs of disease	K Maintaining personal fitness	L Having rich and varied friendships
M	N Being gentle with myself (positive self-talk, nurturing self-care)	O Restricting cholesterol intake
P Wearing a seat belt	Q Having someone I can share my deepest thoughts and feelings with	R Avoiding the traditional health care system whenever possible
S Maintaining a positive outlook; embracing opportunities to grow from life's challenges	T Mobility, flexibility and freedom to engage in demanding physical activity	U Searching out stimulating and new ideas
V Informed use of health care professionals	W Engaging in refreshing relaxation and play	X

156 ASSERTIVE CONSUMER

This exercise empowers individuals to express their health care needs assertively, by writing a letter to people or organizations able to address their concerns.

GOALS

To become proactive about personal health care.

To assert health care needs.

GROUP SIZE

Unlimited.

TIME FRAME

40–50 minutes

MATERIALS NEEDED

One **Assertive Consumer Rough Draft** worksheet, blank paper, and list of local resources (compiled by the trainer) for each participant; **World Almanacs**, at least one for each small group; several other reference books with addresses of pertinent organizations.

PROCESS

☞ *In advance, compile a list of local resources, including key medical, social service, consumer protection, and employee assistance providers, as well as health-related government agencies and political representatives at all levels. Check your local library or bookstore for consumer advocacy reference books.*

1) The trainer introduces the topic by asking participants about the characteristics of an assertive consumer.

   ✔ Think about someone whom you would describe as an assertive consumer. What are the characteristics of this person?

   ✔ How would you describe this individual's attitude toward herself and others?

   ✔ What are some examples of assertive consumer actions that this person has taken?

2) The trainer weaves group responses into a short chalktalk summarizing the characteristics of an assertive consumer.

- **Assertive consumers are proactive rather than reactive.** They do not wait for something bad to happen before they take action. These individuals are thoughtful about what *could* happen, or what *needs to* happen. They anticipate problems, educate themselves about a product or service, learn their rights, and become familiar with resources available to help with these concerns.

- **Assertive consumers demonstrate respect for themselves and others.** They do not act out of righteous indignation, not do they aggressively attack or blame their opponents. Instead they tell the truth without blame or judgment. They express their opinions and allow others to express theirs. Assertive consumers maintain their integrity, as they pursue their goals of clear communication and fair play.

- **Assertive consumers are open to compromise.** Unless their integrity is at stake, assertive people look for compromise. In this way, conflicts are resolved by each person's getting some of what they want.

- **Assertive consumers use learned skills.** People are not born assertive. We learn these skills by study, practice, and support from others.

3) The trainer asks participants to form groups of 4–6 people, according to areas of interest in health issues: physical, mental, emotional, spiritual, and relational. He then guides them through a process of asserting their health care needs.

- ➤ Introduce yourself to the group by describing an experience with a health care product or service that was dissatisfying or troublesome to you.

- ➤ After everyone in the group has shared a negative example, go around the group again, this time briefly describing a health product or service that you thought was outstanding.

4) The trainer solicits examples of disappointing and outstanding experiences, comments on the variety, and categorizes similar situations by type.

- **Rights.** Many situations will involve violation of, challenge to, or protection of human, personal, or civil rights. Stereotyping, discrimination, and offensive behavior or images are common examples.

- **Information.** Many of our best or worst interactions with health care products or services relate to information: inadequate or plentiful, misleading or accurate, important or trivial. False advertising, conflicting opinions, and incomplete instructions are extremely frustrating.

● **Quality of Service or Product.** The timeliness, attentiveness, respectfulness, thoroughness, and efficacy of service are top concerns of consumers. We are also looking for products that do what their descriptions claim.

5) The trainer invites participants to identify several additional opportunities for assertive action for whole person well-being.

➤ Take a sheet of blank paper and use it to keep track of situations or incidents that have affected your well-being as we consider a wide variety of possible areas of concern.

☞ *Give several specific examples in each area as you go along (eg, invasion of privacy during a medical procedure, inadequate ventilation in the workplace, etc).*

➤ Have you had any experiences with **physical** health care products or services that deserved commendation or complaint?

➤ Jot down any examples that come to mind in the areas of medical or dental care, nutrition, exercise, disabilities, alcohol, tobacco, drugs, personal safety, etc.

➤ Include a quick note about who was involved and how you felt.

➤ Have you had any experiences with **mental health** care products or services that were disappointing or outstanding?

➤ Do you know someone who has been denied mental health services? Have you been disappointed or pleased with the quality of counseling service? Do you have any issues around a psychiatric hospitalization or use of medications? What about informed consent? Or services available in the schools?

➤ Record any mental health concerns, including a few details about the situation and people involved.

➤ What about the **spiritual** domain of well-being? How satisfied have you been with the care of your soul?

➤ Have you been subject to judgmental or shaming experiences with a religious group? Or affirmed by inclusive language? Or inspired by a ceremony or pastoral care? What positive or negative examples come to mind when you think about the religious/spiritual dimension?

➤ Write down any examples that come to mind.

➤ What about your **work** environment?

➤ Has your employer taken pains to provide benefits that support you and your family? Is the corporate culture tolerant of excess overtime or unsafe working conditions or discrimination or harassment?

➤ Note any examples of praiseworthy or objectionable practices in your workplace.

6) The trainer solicits ideas from participants on appropriate places for assertive consumers to direct complaints or testimonials, and fills in the gaps as necessary, by noting that participants could write:

Person in **authority** on this issue (employer, committee member, board member, or others who have decision-making powers).

Editors of a magazine involved with the issue.

Media sources—TV, newspaper (letter to the editor, publisher).

Influential people—celebrities, board members of a company, producers of a TV/radio station.

Politicians—local, state, and national level.

Associations related to the issue (American Medical Association).

Licensing boards of hospitals, professional groups, and programs.

Special interest groups—MADD (Mothers Against Drunk Driving).

Other **elected officials** (judges, sheriff, school board members).

County or state **health department**.

Producer of a product.

Store which sells the product.

Insurance companies.

Consumer protection agencies.

Schools, churches, and social service agencies.

7) The trainer announces that group members will be practicing assertive consumer skills by drafting a letter of complaint or testimonial about a health care service or product.

➤ Take the time now to look over the list of examples and think about the health care product or service that you want to write about and where you want to direct your comments.

8) When group members have identified the topic and recipient of their letters, the trainer distributes **Assertive Consumer Rough Draft** worksheets and blank paper, then offers some guidelines for assertive communication in a brief chalktalk.

● **Assertiveness is behavior that enables persons to act in their best interest**, stand up for themselves without undue anxiety, and exercise personal rights without denying the rights of others. What is in your best interest? What are your honest feelings about this product or service? What are your rights and the rights of others involved? Use these questions as a guide for writing your letter.

● **Write with descriptive, not judgmental words**, using the first person "I" to state your opinion and feelings. For example write, "I felt shocked and offended when you accused me of faking pain to collect insurance benefits," instead of, "You were obnoxious and rude."

● **Clearly state what type of response you want** from the individual or organization that you are writing, and indicate the time frame in which you want to receive this response ("I would like a written apology from you before our next appointment on June 30, 1995" or "I would like you to support this legislation by voting for it in the November primary.")

9) The trainer gives instructions for writing the letter.

➤ This letter is not about unfinished business in your personal lives, or for therapeutic healing of old wounds. Your letter should be business-like, concerning issues about which you have passion but can maintain a non-judgmental, respectful attitude toward others in-volved.

➤ Keeping your choosen product or service incident clearly in mind, use your worksheet to direct your letter to the proper recipient, describe what happened in detail, identify who was affected by this product or service and how they were affected, acknowledge how you feel about the situation, and assert what you want now.

➤ Use the next 10–15 minutes to write your letter.

➢ Use your worksheet as a rough draft.

➢ Consult with other members of your group if you want help.

➢ Write your final draft on blank paper.

☞ *Give each group one or more local resource lists, reference books, and* **World Almanacs** *(for researching health care organizations and associations, media addresses, and other consumer information).*

10) When nearly all have finished writing their letters (10–15 minutes), the trainer gives instructions for sharing.

➤ Each person should read your letter aloud to the members of your group.

➤ If you prefer not to read your letter aloud, paraphrase the main idea of your letter—or share whatever you are comfortable sharing with the group.

➤ After each letter reading, other group members should offer sincere praise or words of encouragement for the assertive activities reflected in the letter.

11) The trainer concludes the session with a chalktalk summarizing risks and benefits of asserting health care needs.

● **Assertive behavior does not always yield positive results.** Consider the emotional, political, legal, and psychological effects of your actions. What are the risks to yourself and others? Are you willing to take these risks? Put your letter away for a week, then read it again, and decide whether you want to send it. If there are legal issues involved, it would be wise to consult with an attorney before you commit yourself on paper.

● **Assertive behavior can make a difference.** When you assert yourself, you may gain increased control over products and services affecting your health. You have a greater chance of getting your needs met and for making a real difference in the health care system.

TRAINER'S NOTES

ASSERTIVE CONSUMER ROUGH DRAFT

Date:

Organization/Person:

Address:

Dear:

Here is what happened (or failed to happen):

Who was affected and how:

How I feel about the incident/experience/situation:

What I want:

Closing salutation:

Signature:

157 MEALTIME MEDITATION

In this relaxing, sensory meditation, participants tune into ways to nurture themselves at mealtime.

GOALS

To relax before mealtime.

To recognize bodily signals of hunger.

GROUP SIZE

Unlimited. Easily adapted for individual use.

TIME FRAME

10–15 minutes

MATERIALS NEEDED

Mealtime Meditation script; soothing background music to accompany the meditation (optional).

PROCESS

☞ *This Process is most effective just before a meal or refreshment break.*

1) The trainer gives a warm-up chalktalk on mealtime as an opportunity for self-care.

   ● **Hunger is our internal call for nourishment**. Our bodies signal us when we need food or water. When we care for ourselves, we listen to these physical cues and respond accordingly.

   ● **Listening to our bodies is sometimes difficult**. We are bombarded by external cues to eat: tempting food ads; business meetings scheduled at noon; family and friends gathering to socialize and celebrate; fast food lanes offering convenient, inexpensive food; and vending machines with snacks everywhere.

   ● **We often eat for non-physical reasons** including habit, scheduled meals, eating to prevent hunger later in the day, and dependence on the advice of authorities about what, when, and how much to eat.

2) The trainer invites group members to take a quick check on their current level of physical hunger.

> ➤ Take a deep breath, close your eyes, and place your hand on your abdomen. Slowly exhale out your mouth, and continue to breathe deeply, in and out while allowing yourself to relax.

> ➤ Focus your attention inward, and listen to signals of hunger in your stomach.

> ➤ Decide how hungry you are on a scale of 1–10, with 1 being starved, 5 being satisfied, and 10 being stuffed.

> ➤ When you have rated your hunger level for this moment, open your eyes and return your attention to your surroundings.

3) The trainer polls the group on their hunger levels (How many 10s? How many 0s?) and clarifies any questions about the scale.

4) The trainer invites participants to join in a guided imagery experience designed to help people relax and tune in to their body needs before a meal.

> ☞ *Make sure your voice and the music are audible to all. Encourage individuals who have trouble hearing to move closer to you.*

5) The trainer starts the music and reads the **Mealtime Meditation** script.

> ☞ *Be sure to read in a clear, natural, expressive voice, allowing plenty of time for pauses indicated on the script. Practice reading the meditation beforehand, ideally on audiotape so you can hear yourself and modify your tempo or tone.*

6) When the mediation is finished, the trainer encourages everyone to have a wonderful, nourishing meal that sends a strong message of love and care to themselves.

VARIATIONS

> ■ *Lunch Duets* (**Wellness 2**, p 58), *Consciousness-Raising Diet* (**Wellness 3**, p 60), *Eating Under Stress* (**Stress 5**, p 76), and the *Anti-Stress Coffee Break* (**Stress 5**, p 113) combine well with this meditation in a longer workshop focused on eating issues.

MEALTIME MEDITATION Script

Take a moment now to relax . . .
Settle back in a comfortable chair . . .
and allow your body to rest against the surface of the chair . . .

Take a deep breath . . . close your eyes . . .
and fill yourself with air . . .
Then let it out . . . slowly and easily . . .
blowing softly out of your mouth . . .
Breathe in again . . . deeply through your nose . . .
filling your lungs from bottom to top . . .
Then slowly . . . softly . . . let that breath go . . .
relaxing and calming your body . . .

☞ *Pause 5 seconds.*

Continue to breathe deeply . . . slowly and easily . . .
responding to your body's call for air . . .
Filling the exact needs of your body with each breath . . .
Not too much . . . not too little . . .
Each breath brings the perfect amount . . .

☞ *Pause 5 seconds.*

Imagine your body's need for food . . .
and your response to this call . . .
It's easy and natural . . . like breathing . . .
responding to your hunger . . .
giving your body the nourishment it needs . . .
Not too much . . . not too little . . .
but just the right amount for you . . .

Notice the rhythm of your breathing . . .
as you consider your need for food at this very moment . . .
Focus on the feelings in your body . . .
as you allow yourself to listen to hunger signals . . .
which may be vibrating from your abdomen . . .
softly stirring, rumbling, or roaring . . .

Notice these sounds and sensations . . .
Listen to the voice of your body . . .

☞ *Pause 5 seconds.*

Perhaps it is quiet . . . satisfied . . . resting . . .

Images of non-physical hungers may drift in and out of your awareness . . .

You might find your thoughts drifting off . . .
to a pleasant fantasy . . . or distractions from your day . . .
If this happens . . . simply notice these thoughts and sensations . . .
as you let them pass through your awareness . . .
Whatever you are doing . . . wherever you are going . . .
whatever you are feeling . . .
is exactly right for you at this moment . . .
You are wise . . . and your body is wise . . .

You can trust yourself to know what to do for yourself . . .
and how to do it . . .
You are your body's best friend . . .

Notice the sensations in your mouth . . .
Tune in to the kind of food that your mouth wants to taste . . .

☞ *Pause 5 seconds.*

Does it crave a soft, creamy food . . . or a hard and crunchy texture?
Does it want something hot . . . or cold . . . liquid . . . or solid?

Perhaps images of food will pass through your mind . . .
Allow them to move through your awareness . . . simply noticing them . . .
You can trust yourself to make wise choices . . .
knowing how to feed your body what it needs . . .
to stay healthy . . . active . . . and feeling good . . .

You can trust your body to tell you what it needs . . .
and you can trust yourself to satisfy these needs . . .

☞ *Pause 10 seconds.*

As you continue to relax and explore your hunger . . .
you are aware of your human needs . . .
and you accept and love yourself . . .
You are worthwhile . . .
and you deserve the life-sustaining nutrients of a good meal . . .

Let yourself have exactly what you want . . . and the pleasure of eating it . . .
Food is not your only pleasure . . .
so you can relax and enjoy your meal fully . . .
trusting that you will not overeat . . .

You can give yourself exactly what you need . . .
no more . . . no less . . .

©1995 Whole Person Press 210 W Michigan Duluth MN 55802　　　(800) 247-6789

Eating is like breathing . . . natural and easy . . .
You will stop when you have had enough . . .

Focus now on the kind of food you are wanting . . .
and the amount that you think you need . . .
Pay attention to these ideas and images . . .
and trust yourself to use them wisely . . .

☞ *Pause 10 seconds.*

As you prepare to return to the present . . .
know that you can take this knowledge with you . . .
when you go for your next meal . . .

You can continue this feeling of relaxation . . .
and confidence in yourself . . . and your body . . .
You are your own best friend.

When you are ready . . .
slowly open your eyes . . . and return to the present . . .
feeling relaxed . . . calm . . .
and connected to your body . . .

158 HEALTHY EXERCISE

This short video and self-analysis process stimulates, inspires, and empowers participants to seek the health benefits of an exercise they can enjoy.

GOALS

To learn about the effects of exercise on overall health, longevity, and risk factors for disease.

To assess personal exercise patterns and confront barriers to regular exercise.

To choose an enjoyable fitness activity.

GROUP SIZE

Unlimited.

TIME FRAME

20–60 minutes

MATERIALS NEEDED

A VHS VCR and monitor; *Healthy Exercise* videotape (20 min), third of six in a series on **Making Healthy Choices**, available from Whole Person Associates, 210 W Michigan St, Duluth, MN 55802. 1-800-247-6787. FAX 218-727-0505. (Purchase cost $95.00, includes **Leader Guide** and five colorful **Skill Building Guides** for participants. Additional **Skill Building Guides**, with supplemental content material, intriguing worksheets, process instructions, and summaries of the videotapes, are available at an attractive discount.)

PROCESS

☞ *This complete process is outlined in detail in the Skill Building Guides and Leader Guide that accompany the Healthy Eating video.*

1) The trainer provides a warm-up chalktalk on the benefits of exercise and invites participants to reflect upon their current level of physical activity by answering thought-provoking questions in a worksheet.

2) The trainer asks participants to introduce themselves and other group members and briefly share what they wrote.

3) The trainer plays the videotape.

☞ *This twenty-minute video asks a variety of people—both experts and everyday folks—about the benefits of exercise, three types of physical activity important for any exercise program, how much exercise is enough, the barriers to activity, and steps for overcoming these obstacles. It also includes a three-minute closing relaxation sequence.*

4) The trainer challenges participants to evaluate their current exercise patterns, and write an essay on assigned topics related to their exercise patterns.

5) The trainer instructs participants to share their essays with one another.

6) The trainer invites participants to examine their excuses for not exercising and then to imagine ways to overcome these barriers and create an exercise program they would enjoy.

7) Participants complete an **Activity Analysis** to discover activities they think would be fun.

8) The trainer offers practical hints for getting started, and then encourages group members to write a plan for developing an exercise program they can do and enjoy.

9) The trainer guides participants through a small group sharing process, to bring closure to the session.

10) The trainer ends the session by advising participants to take a walk, pointing out the benefits of this easy, inexpensive activity in a closing chalktalk.

VARIATIONS

■ Use the video tape alone for a 15–20 minute information session, or expand it to fill a longer period by allowing more time for participants to complete worksheets and engage in discussion.

*Based on the **Making Healthy Choices** video series (Duluth MN: Whole Person Press, 1995).*

159 IMAGERY FOR A HEALTHY HEART

This directed daydream technique evens out blood pressure and helps maintain open arteries and a strong, healthy heart.

GOALS

To practice visualization and sensory imaging techniques.

To learn a practical technique for maintaining a healthy circulatory system.

TIME FRAME

10–15 minutes

MATERIALS NEEDED

Imagery for a Healthy Heart script; CD or cassette player and slow, flowing relaxation music (optional).

PROCESS

☞ *Imagery is not a substitute for professional medical care. Encourage participants to get regular checkups and follow their doctor's orders. Guided imagery should be used as a supplement to prescribed preventive or care regimens.*

This exercise assumes participants have prior knowledge of the risks and dynamics of coronary artery disease as well as a good understanding of appropriate strategies for regaining/maintaining a healthy circulatory system.

1) The trainer introduces the exercise with a brief chalktalk on the guided imagery and how it can be used to enhance well-being.

- **Guided imagery could be called a directed daydream**, a process in which you use the power of your imagination to help your mind and body perform at optimum capacity, stay strong, or heal from trauma when needed.

- **Guided imagery is a powerful whole person tool for health** and healing, since our bodies interpret sensory images from the imagination in the same way as sensory data from real life experience. Just as unhealthy images can make us sick, healthful images can positively impact our well-being.

● Modern scientific research is accruing compelling data on the health engineering capability of our imaginations. Not only is guided imagery great for relaxation, stress reduction, and enhancement, these techniques have also been demonstrated to:

reduce aversive responses to chemotherapy.

increase the number of circulating white cells.

increase the level of T receptor cells.

increase immune function.

decrease (or increase!) allergic reaction.

positively impact depression and acne.

speed up postsurgical wound healing.

reduce the need for pain medication in postsurgical, orthopedic, and severe burn patients.

● **Imagery can help keep you healthy.** Research also suggests that coronary artery disease is sometimes reversible without surgery when individuals regularly practice guided imagery routines that are designed to even out blood pressure, open arteries, and encourage a strong heart.

2) The trainer invites participants to try the imagining process for a healthy heart, reading the **Imagery for a Healthy Heart** script.

☞ *Don't rush! People need time to allow the images to form. You may want to respond to potential resistance up front by suggesting that folks suspend their judgement and try to stay with the flow of the images, even if nothing seems to be happening.*

3) The trainer invites comments from the group, and uses these to clarify issues related to guided imagery and/or heart disease.

IMAGERY FOR A HEALTHY HEART Script

Please try to position yourself as comfortably as you can . . .
shifting your weight so that you're allowing your body
to feel fully supported . . .
See if you can arrange it so your head, neck, and spine are straight.

And just taking a deep, full, cleansing breath . . .
inhaling as fully as your comfortably can . . . (pause) . . .
and exhaling fully . . . (pause) . . .

And once more . . .
breathing in and sending the warm energy of the breath
to any part of your body that's tense or sore or tight . . .
and releasing the tension with the exhale . . .
so you can feel your breath going to all the tight, tense places . . .
loosening and softening them . . .
and then gathering up all the tension and breathing it out . . .
so that more and more, you can feel safe and comfortable . . .
relaxed and easy . . .
watching the cleansing action of the breath . . .
with friendly but detached awareness . . .

And any unwelcome thoughts that come to mind . . .
those, too, can be sent out with the breath . . .
released with the exhale . . .
so that for just a moment, the mind is empty . . .
for just a split second, it is free and clear space,
and you are blessed with stillness . . .

And any emotions that are rocking around in there . . .
those, too, are noted and acknowledged . . .
and sent out with the breath . . .
so that your emotional self can be still and quiet . . .
like a lake with no ripples . . .

And now, gently allowing yourself to turn your attention inward . . .
focusing inside for just this next while . . .
to see how your body feels . . .

And turning your attention, if you would,
to the subtle sensation of your blood, moving through your body . . .
perhaps feeling its steady warmth . . . moving all through you . . .
perhaps hearing it vibrate and hum as it moves along . . .

or maybe seeing the exquisite, intricate pattern of veins and arteries . . .
wide and powerful at your center . . .
and delicate and filigreed at your outermost edges . . .

So just taking a few moments to acknowledge your remarkable
system of circulation . . . so strong and steady . . . (pause) . . .

And aware that the blood moving through your body . . .
so steadily and easily . . .
seems to have an exquisite intelligence of its own . . .
a built-in ability to repair and heal everything it touches . . .
and you can feel it . . . softly and easily rolling along . . .
gently expanding the vessels as it goes . . .
making more room for the rich supplies that it brings . . .

And softening the walls of the arteries as it moves along . . .
making them into more flexible, enduring stuff . . .
keeping the inner lining slick and smooth and shiny . . .
with no place for debris to cling to it . . .

And strengthening and replenishing the arteries' weaker spots . . .
should there be any . . .
and perhaps there are none . . .
but in case there are . . .
shoring up any thin places along the walls . . .
as the rich, steady supply continues to roll along . . .
like a gentle river . . . rich and full and nourishing . . .
bringing everything that's needed to fortify the walls . . .
safely and easily . . .
as constant and steady as the earth rolling through the heavens . . .

And sensing how the steady flow . . .
gradually reduces whatever small collection of unwanted debris
might have begun to gather here and there along the sides . . .
gently and safely eroding
whatever tiny buildup that might have accumulated in the lining . . .
perhaps some small, fatty streaks . . .
or possibly a few older, more crusty places . . .
gradually and safely eroding them . . .
wearing them down to smooth, clean slickness . . .
safely expanding each vessel, big or small . . .
the wide, powerful ones around the heart . . .
in the neck . . . and shoulders . . . and thighs . . .
and the smaller ones that make up the whole miraculous network . . .
down to the tiniest, laciest filigree of capillaries in the fingers and toes . . .

Opening the narrower places . . .
and allowing for an even, steady flow . . .
gentle and strong in the wide, smooth, soft arteries . . .

And dissolving any matter in the bloodstream itself . . .
turning any beginnings of clotting into tiny microdots . . .
and dispersing them, safely and easily . . .

A gentle, steady river . . .
feeding the hungry tissue along its banks . . .
And just sensing how the sugar and nutrients in the blood
leach out into the surrounding field of tissue . . .
soaked up by the hungry cells . . .
in a steady, continuous supply . . .

And feeling the hungry tissue respond . . .
sensing the cells plump up to full strength from this steady, generous source . . .
as new life and energy return . . .
organ and muscle and bone rebuilding . . .
as cells replace themselves . . .
and the body charges up with strength and purpose . . .
remembering its power and vitality . . .

And so . . . feeling all through your body
the penetrating warmth and power of this awareness . . .
grateful for your capacity for healing and renewal . . .
strong and steady and resilient . . .

And so, once again . . .
feeling yourself in your surroundings . . .
taking a deep, full breath . . . gently and with soft eyes . . .
coming back into the room whenever you are ready . . .
knowing you are better for this . . .

And so you are . . .

*This script is one of several powerful visualizations for well-being in Belleruth Naparstek's book, **Staying Well with Guided Imagery** (New York: Warner Books, 1994).*

160 SEVENTH INNING STRETCH

In this invigorating exercise, participants combine fantasy with systematic relaxation skills to stretch each muscle group in the body.

GOALS

To relax and revitalize the body and mind.

To connect actions in a relaxation sequence with memorable imagery cues.

GROUP SIZE

Unlimited.

TIME FRAME

5–10 minutes

MATERIALS NEEDED

Seventh Inning Stretch handout.

PROCESS

1) The trainer introduces the stretch with a brief chalktalk about stress and relaxation.

   ● **Stress is a physiological process.** Whether or not we are consciously aware of the process, when we are under stress, our muscles tense, and our nervous, cardiovascular, and endocrine systems go into overdrive. Tense muscles can interfere with other primary functions such as blood pressure, digestion, mental processing, and emotional arousal.

   ● **Relaxation is our body's natural antidote for stress.** When we systematically relax our muscles, the fibers **lengthen**, and give up their stranglehold on other viral body tissues. When we are relaxed, our body uses energy with greater efficiency and we are less prone to a startle reflex when confronted with stressors.

   ● During the 1930s Dr Edmund Jacobsen developed a technique for helping people learn how to relax at will, by deliberately tensing and then releasing muscles in all parts of the body. This **systematic progressive relaxation** is one of the most effective skills we can learn for managing stress and its side effects.

● **Imagery can enhance the potential of relaxation.** By combining imagery with muscle tension-and-relaxation sequences, we can amplify the relaxation benefits. Imagery can also transform a potentially dreary self-care chore into a playful activity, while it helps us remember the proper sequence.

2) The trainer invites participants to stand and join in a **Seventh Inning Stretch**.

3) The trainer gives general instructions and then leads the group through the sequence of fifteen steps outlined in the **Seventh Inning Stretch** handout.

➤ Make yourself as comfortable as possible.

➢ Spread out so you have some elbow room.

➢ Remove your glasses, if you wish, and loosen any restrictive collars or belts.

➤ As you try each movement in sequence, pay attention to your physical sensations. Notice the contrast between muscles in a state of tension and a state of relaxation.

VARIATIONS

■ Introduce the stretches early in the session. Then repeat the whole sequence as a closing energizer and reminder. Sprinkle stretch breaks throughout a longer workshop, highlighting different muscle groups each time.

Submitted by Mary O'Brien Sippel.

SEVENTH INNING STRETCH

For each stretch, try to keep all other muscles relaxed as you concentrate on tensing just the muscles in the specific group. For maximum benefit, exaggerate the movements so your muscles really get a workout before you relax. Alternate 10–20 seconds of muscle tension/ stretching with a similar period of relaxation before moving to the next muscle group. Pay attention to the different sensations of tension and relaxation.

1) Imagine there is a fly on your forehead or nose. Scrunch up and wiggle the muscles of your face as you struggle to get that fly to move.

2) Close your lips and imagine you are pushing a ball of air from side to side in your mouth, between your cheeks, behind, then in front of, your teeth.

3) Imagine you are chewing a big bite of something hard and chewy.

4) Imagine yourself as a turtle, hiding in your shell, with your head tucked in and your shoulders straining up to protect you.

5) Imagine your are inflating a balloon in your abdomen, blowing your belly further and further out . . . until finally the balloon pops, and your chest collapses along with your abdomen.

6) Imagine you are trying to sneak through a narrow opening in a picket fence. Make yourself as tall and skinny as possible so you can inch your way through without getting stuck.

7) Imagine you are squeezing a big, juicy lemon in each hand, kneading and squeezing it tighter and tighter so you can extract every drop of juice.

8) Imagine your hands are starfish, stretching out in search of plankton, pulsing with the rhythm of the tide.

9) Imagine you are picking luscious fruit from a branch you can barely reach. Stand on your tiptoes, with most of your weight on your left foot as you stretch out and up with your right arm to reach the fruit. Relax. And then stretch up again with your left hand, balancing on your right toes.

10) Imagine you are out in your driveway with a brand new hula hoop, trying to set a world record. Rotate your hips and pelvis and trunk in rhythm to keep the hoop moving.

11) Imagine your upper legs are filling with concrete that is quickly solidifying. Make your legs as dense and tight as a concrete pillar from hip to toe.

12) Imagine you are pulling on a pair of tight, long socks or boots. Start with your toes and slowly pull all the way up to your knee or thigh, stretching your whole leg and foot. Relax. Repeat with the opposite leg.

13) Imagine you are a duck, walking on your heels, with your toes curled under.

14) Imagine your foot is a helicopter propeller rotating round and round your ankle, preparing for takeoff. Relax. Then rev up your other foot and ankle.

15) Imagine you are in bed at night and have just heard a noise downstairs. Tense every muscle in your body as you shrink in terror or prepare to jump the intruder.

161 MENTAL HEALTH INDEX

Participants define mental health, learn about six common mental health problems, assess their own mental health, and discuss strategies for caring for themselves and others when problems occur.

GOALS

To promote mental health.

To increase awareness of common mental health problems, symptoms, and treatments.

To provide an introduction for EAP services.

GROUP SIZE

Unlimited.

TIME FRAME

30–45 minutes

MATERIALS NEEDED

Mental Health Check-Up worksheet for each participant; newsprint; a list of EAP and mental health resources in your community.

PROCESS

1) The trainer introduces the topic by telling the group that psychoanalyst Sigmund Freud defined mental health as "the capacity to work and play." He asks participants to generate their own definitions of **mental health**, and writes all ideas on a newsprint.

2) The trainer then asks participants what **mental illness** is, and writes the group definitions on a second newsprint. He challenges participants to think about all of the things that fall between the two extremes of health and illness, leading group members to recognize shades of grey and to view mental health on a continuum from very well to very ill.

   ☞ *Remind participants that mental health is a dynamic state of being, and that all people move back and forth on the continuum at different times of their lives.*

3) The trainer uses the group definitions and self-assessment as a springboard for a chalktalk describing six mental health problems that com-
monly touch peoples lives.

- **Adjustment problems** are reactions to stressful life changes that
  require adaptation or adjustment on our part (eg, moving, starting a
  new job, building a house, grieving multiple losses, caring for a
  chronically ill relative or family member). Such stresses are problem-
  atic when they cause a temporary upset in our ability to function at
  work or school, in social activities, or in relationships with others.
  Adjustment problems usually last for no more than six months. People
  going through such adjustment difficulties may be emotional, irritable, anxious, moderately depressed, less effective at work, and
  generally out-of-sorts.

- People who suffer from **anxiety or panic problems** find themselves
  worrying excessively or unrealistically for a period of six months or
  longer. They may experience a variety of symptoms: tension, restless-
  ness, fatigue, shortness of breath, palpitations or accelerated heart
  rate, dry mouth, sweating, dizziness, abnormal distress, frequent
  urination, feeling keyed up or on edge, difficulty concentrating or
  "mind going blank" because of anxiety, trouble sleeping, or irritabil-
  ity. Some may have panic attacks which are sudden unexpected
  periods of intense fear or discomfort. These problems may be short-
  term or long term, depending on a variety of circumstances: family
  history, life stressors, coping skills, and resources available.

- **Post-Traumatic Stress Disorder** is a form of anxiety experienced by
  people who have experienced a traumatic event that is outside the
  range of usual human experiences—war, physical assault (including
  sexual abuse and rape), natural disasters, serious threat or harm to a
  loved one, accidents, and witnessing tragic events. Symptoms include
  recurrent and intrusive distressing memories of the event, flashbacks
  (reliving the event), and intense psychological distress when confronted with reminders of the event. People experiencing trauma
  often feel disconnected from others, unable to feel loving feelings,
  and uninterested in their routine activities. Usually these severe
  reactions develop soon after the trauma, are intense for a period of one
  or two months, and gradually diminish over several years.

- **Family problems.** A family therapist once said that a good measure
  of family health is whether anyone takes out the garbage. When
  families become dysfunctional, routine chores may not get done.
  Something is not working. People are not talking to each other;
  tension has reached an exploding point. Arguments, absences, power

struggles, abuse, and other signs of stress may be obvious. Unless these problems are recognized and treated, the capacity of everyone in the family—adults and children—to function at work or school is affected.

● **Alcohol, drug and gambling addictions.** Chemical dependency counselors often define addiction as "continuing to use the addictive substance even when the user is experiencing multiple problems as a result of this use." Continuing to drink when doctors have warned of heart and liver disease, continuing to use drugs after repeated job losses, continuing to gamble in spite of mounting debts and legal problems, all speak of trouble. Addictions affect the mental health of all the people who live with, or love and care for, the addicted person. Spouses and children of chemically dependent people may suffer anxiety, depression, and other mental health problems.

● **Depression.** Depression is the world's number one public health problem, according to Dr. David Burns of the University of Pennsylvania's School of Medicine. Symptoms of depression are persistent depressed mood, loss of interest or pleasure in nearly all activities, significant weight loss or gain, insomnia or excessive sleep, fatigue or loss of energy, feelings of worthlessness or excessive guilt, inability to concentrate, and recurring thoughts of death. When these kinds of symptoms are present for more that two weeks, it is important to seek professional help.

Most of us will not need professional help for the kinds of depression we experience from time to time. Unhealed grief from a series of losses, being a perfectionist, trying to live up to other people's expectations, can all lead to depression. But supportive relationships, using our personal powers, and physical activities like walking, can bring healing for these pains.

4) The trainer distributes copies of the **Mental Health Check-Up** worksheet to each participant, and encourages them to assess their own current mental health. He suggests that they view any "yes" answers as signals of a need for change, problem-solving, or getting help.

5) The trainer facilitates a group discussion on the process for maintaining or regaining mental health.

☞ *For each issue, record responses from the group and post them. Be ready with examples to prime the pump.*

● Prevention is the best care.

✔ What can you do to prevent mental health problems?

● Once you notice a problem, self-care is the treatment of choice.

✔ What are some self-care strategies and options for mental health problems?

● When self-care efforts don't work, it's time to seek the assistance of self-help groups and professionals.

✔ What can you do when your self-care efforts don't work to restore your equilibrium?

☞ *If you have a list of mental health resources for your community or employee group, pass these out now.*

6) The trainer concludes with a chalktalk providing guidelines for knowing when and how to seek professional help for mental health concerns.

● The American Association for Marriage and Family Therapy recommends you consider consulting a mental health professional if you experience any of the following symptoms:

Persistent feelings of dissatisfaction with marriage or family life.
Problems with a child's behavior, school adjustment, or performance.
Sexual problems or concerns.
Inexplainable fatigue.
Difficulties talking with your fiancé, spouse, child, parents, other family members, friends or co-workers.
Feeling of loneliness, moodiness, depression, failure, anxiety.
The need for tranquilizers, energizers, or sleeping aids.
Family stress due to repeated illnesses or illness in which stress plays a major role.
Problems with alcohol, drugs, or gambling.
Repeated financial difficulties.
Difficulty in setting or reaching goals.
Drastic weight fluctuations or irregular eating patterns.
Work difficulties, frequent job changes, problems with co-workers.
Unmanageable anger, hostility, or violence.

● There are many possible options in choosing professional help for mental health issues: clergy, social workers, child psychologists, family therapists, psychiatrists, guidance counselors, chemical dependency counselors, chaplains, group counselors, nurse practitioners, and other professionals are available for help with a crisis.

● When you do seek professional help, inquire about the credentials (experience, training, and professional licenses) of your counselor. Ask about your client rights and make sure you understand the nature of the therapy you are starting, as well as the cost.

MENTAL HEALTH CHECK-UP

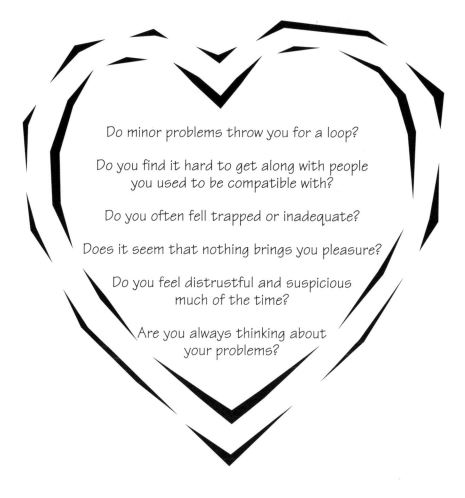

Do minor problems throw you for a loop?

Do you find it hard to get along with people
you used to be compatible with?

Do you often fell trapped or inadequate?

Does it seem that nothing brings you pleasure?

Do you feel distrustful and suspicious
much of the time?

Are you always thinking about
your problems?

Source: National Mental Health Association

162 SEVEN WAYS OF KNOWING

Participants explore all seven of their intelligences with this creative, affirming tribute to differing gifts.

GOALS

To expand understanding of multimodal intelligence.

To identify personal strengths and problem solving style.

To practice strategies for enhancing intelligences.

GROUP SIZE

Unlimited.

TIME FRAME

60–90 minutes. Easy to modify for shorter or longer time frame.

MATERIALS NEEDED

Seven Ways of Knowing worksheets; Hi-lighters in variety of colors, one for each participant; large wall calendar or overhead transparency that shows the entire year; signs or posters identifying each group by day of the week, type of intelligence, and group task (for *Steps 11* and *12*); large sheets of newsprint and markers, masking tape, writing materials and paper for group projects.

PROCESS

☞ *This exercise requires more preparation than most. Make sure you have all materials ready in advance, including signs.*

1) The trainer begins by posing a question to the group.

   ✔ How many of you would like to be more intelligent?

      ☞ *Comment on the response, promising that everyone will automatically increase their intelligence today.*

2) The trainer solicits ideas from the group on what they believe intelligence is.

   ☞ *Affirm all answers as being potentially part of intelligence.*

3) The trainer uses these responses as illustrations for an introductory chalktalk on the nature of intelligence.

● Since the early 1900s, when Binet developed a test to measure intelligence, people have been labeled and categorized (and possibly terrorized) by an impersonal number that is supposed to represent a measure of comparative intellectual capability.

● Although IQ was never intended as a complete measure of potential, educators, psychologists, and the general public embraced the concept wholeheartedly and most of us have been brainwashed to believe that it's the only measure that counts.

● Today we understand intelligence from a more universal perspective. Current research into the nature of intelligence indicates that intelligence is a much more complex quality than originally conceptualized. Dr. Howard Gardner and his team of researchers at Harvard define intelligence as the ability to solve the problems that face us and produce things that are of value to our culture. This definition leaves much more room for us to affirm our own intelligence as well as that of others.

○ **Intelligence is not a static quality.** We have the ability to enhance and amplify our intelligence. No matter what your age or ability level, you can improve your mental functioning. We can also teach others to be more intelligent.

○ **There are many important forms of intelligence**, involving the entire brain/mind system that are not measured by traditional IQ tests. As with other human qualities, some folks have more natural gifts in some forms of intelligence than others—or at least have exercised some more than others.

○ Although we have different forms of intelligence, when confronted with a problem to solve or project to accomplish, **all aspects of intelligence work together to accomplish the goal**.

4) The trainer invites participants to participate in a one question IQ test.

➤ Pat and Chris are walking together down the street. Pat's step is two-thirds that of Chris. They want to keep walking together.

How many step will they each have to take before their left feet hit the ground at the same time again.?

➤ Take one minute to solve this problem in any way you can.

➤ As you work, notice what you are doing to get an answer.

🖙 *Pay attention to the group as they work, noting examples of strategies illustrating the multimodal intelligences.*

5) The trainer asks for solutions (the answer is Pat = 6 steps, Chris = 4 steps), solicits examples of how participants tackled the problem solving process and weaves them into a chalktalk on multiple intelligence problem solving.

● Some people will close their eyes and imagine the pair walking. Some instinctively grab paper and pencil to draw the figures or footsteps, others will quickly construct an algebraic equation to solve the problem. Some may use fingers or hands to tap out the rhythm of the steps. Others simply sit and meditate, waiting for the answer to arrive spontaneously. And, or course, some can't resist discussing the problem.

☞ *Ask if any one was tempted to get up and step it out with a partner.*

● Although we might typically define the most intelligent person as the one who used the correct algebraic formula, all of these very different strategies successfully solved the problem correctly.

6) The trainer distribute **Seven Ways of Knowing** worksheets and invites participants to consider their problem-solving style.

● Each of us has a style of approaching problems that seems natural to us. It could be a strategy that has worked well in the past. Or one that feels comfortable. Or one that life has taught us to trust. Or one that seems to fit our personality.

● Dr. Howard Gardner, the researcher from Harvard who provided the concept of multiple intelligence, identified seven distinct ways that we learn and know about reality. He also suspects that there are other intelligences we have not yet identified and documented.

● Teacher, educator, and curriculum developer Dr. David Lazear has expanded Gardner's concept, calling these multiple intelligences the **Seven Ways of Knowing**, and details strategies for developing strategies for developing intelligence in each area.

☞ *Encourage participants to take notes as you describe the seven way of knowing.*

● **Verbal/Linguistic Intelligence** is responsible for the production of language and all the complex possibilities that follow, including poetry, humor, story-telling, grammar, metaphors, similes, abstract reasoning, symbolic thinking, conceptual patterning, reading and writing.

This intelligence can be seen in such people as poets, playwrights, storytellers, novelists, public speakers, and comedians.

- **Logical/Mathematical Intelligence** is most often associated with what we call "scientific thinking" or inductive reasoning, although deductive thought processes are also involved. This intelligence involves the capacity to recognize patterns, work with abstract symbols (such as numbers and geometric shapes), and discern relationships and/or see connections between separate and distinct pieces of information.

  This intelligence can be seen in such people as scientists, computer programmers, accountants, lawyers, bankers, and, of course, mathematicians.

- Unfortunately, these are the only two types of intelligence that we have traditionally measured and valued. Logical/mathematical and verbal/linguistic intelligence provide the basis for most systems of Western education, as well as for all forms of currently existing standardized testing programs.

- **Visual/Spatial Intelligence** deals with such things as the visual arts (including painting, drawing, and sculpture); navigation, map-making, and architecture (which involve the use of space and knowing how to get around in it); and games such as chess (which require the ability to visualize objects from different perspectives and angles). The key sensory base of this intelligence is the sense of sight, but also the ability to form mental images and pictures in the mind.

  This intelligence can be seen in such people as architects, graphic design artists, cartographers, industrial designers, and, of course, producers of the visual arts (painters and sculptors).

- **Body/Kinesthetic Intelligence** is the ability to use the body to express emotion (as in dance and body language), to play a game (as in sports), and to create a new product (as in invention). *Learning by doing* has long been recognized as an important part of education. Our bodies know things our minds don't and can't know in any other way. For example, it is our bodies that know how to ride a bike, roller skate, type, and parallel park a car.

  This intelligence can be seen in such people as actors, athletes, mimes, professional dancers, and inventors.

- **Musical/Rhythmic Intelligence** includes such capacities as the recognition and use of rhythmic and tonal patterns, and sensitivity to sounds from the environment, the human voice, and musical instruments. Many of us learned the alphabet through this intelligence and the *A-B-C song*. Of all forms of intelligence, the *consciousness altering* effect of music and rhythm on the brain is probably the greatest.

This intelligence can be seen in advertising people (those who write catchy jingles to sell a product), professional performance musicians, rock groups, dance bands, composers, and music teachers.

● **Interpersonal Intelligence** involves the ability to work cooperatively with others in a group as well as the ability to communicate, verbally and non-verbally, with other people. It builds on the capacity to notice distinctions among others; for example, contrasts in moods, temperament, motivations, and intentions. In the more advanced forms of this intelligence, one can literally "pass over" into another's perspective and "read" their intentions and desires. One can have genuine empathy for another's feelings, fears, anticipations, and beliefs.

This form of intelligence is usually highly developed in such people as counselors, teachers, therapists, politicians, and religious leaders.

● **Intrapersonal Intelligence** involves knowledge of the internal aspects of the self, such as knowledge of feelings, the range of emotional responses, thinking processes, self-reflection, and a sense of or intuition about spiritual realities. Intrapersonal intelligence allows us to be conscious of our consciousness; that is, to step back from ourselves and watch ourselves as an outside observer. It involves our capacity to experience wholeness and unity, to discern patterns of connection with the larger order of things, to perceive higher states of consciousness, to experience the lure of the future, and to dream of and actualize the possible.

This intelligence can be seen in such people as philosophers, psychiatrists, spiritual counselors and gurus, and cognitive pattern researchers.

7) The trainer polls the group for a how of hands indicating which of these seven intelligences participants used for solving the Pat and Chris problem.

8) The trainer distributes Hi-lighters to the group and asks participants to identify their "natural" intelligence.

➤ In the *left column* Hi-light the **way of knowing** that feels **most natural** and comfortable to you. Which strategy do you typically use for problem solving?

➤ In the *right column* Hi-light for each intelligence those activities you would be likely to engage in.

➤ Now trade markers with a neighbor, so you have a different color, and mark the **knowing strategy** you would **least likely use** in solving a problem.

9) The trainer directs participants to pair up with a neighbor and compare notes.

➤ Share your most natural, comfortable mode of problem-solving.

➤ Describe one example of when you used that strategy effectively.

☞ *Interrupt after 2 minutes.*

➤ Now discuss your least utilized way of knowing.

➤ What stops you from exercising this intelligence more often?

10) The trainer reconvenes the whole group and asks for observations and solicits examples of what inhibited people from using different intelligences.

11) The trainer announces that participants will have an opportunity to exercise one of their seven intelligences in a small group.

➤ In a moment you will divide into groups on the basis of the day of the week your birthday falls this year.

➤ Figure out what day your birthday is this year.

☞ *Put the calendar transparency on the overhead or point out the posted wall calendar.*

➤ Listen to the instructions for all groups. You may want to take notes on their assignments.

➤ Your group's task will also be posted at your meeting place.

➤ **Mondays** will represent *verbal/linguistic* intelligence.

➤ Your task will be to write a serious or humorous poem, story, or speech that celebrates the seven ways of knowing.

➤ **Tuesday**s will represent *logical/mathematical* intelligence.

➤ Your task will be to make up a game to help people remember the multiple intelligences.

➤ **Wednesdays** will represent *visual/spatial* intelligence.

➤ Your task will be to make a mural or poster that conveys the seven ways of knowing.

➤ **Thursdays** will represent the *body/kinesthetic* intelligence.

➤ Your task is to develop a dance you can teach to the others that portrays or demonstrates the seven ways of knowing through body movements and gestures.

➤ **Fridays** will represent the *musical/rhythmic* intelligence.

➤ Your task is to create a song with seven different sounds, rhythms, tunes, or percussion that teaches or demonstrates the seven ways of knowing.

➤ **Saturdays** will represent *interpersonal* intelligence.

   ➤ Your task is to design a small or large group project that includes personal sharing and discussion about the seven ways of knowing.

➤ **Sundays** will represent *intrapersonal* intelligence.

   ➤ Your task is to develop a personal reflection or guided imagery process to help individuals mentally explore their seven ways of knowing.

12) The trainer points out the designated gathering points for the groups and notes that groups will have 20 minutes to finish their tasks.

13) After 20 minutes, the trainer gathers all groups and asks each one in turn to present their creation, beginning with the group whose birthdays fell on today's day of the week.

14) After the gala intelligence demonstration is complete, the trainer invites participants to look once again at their worksheets.

➤ Trade Hi-lighters with a neighbor so you have a different color.

➤ Look through the list of **capacities** in the *middle column*, and Hi-light any aspects of intelligence you would like to develop more fully.

15) In closing, the trainer reviews strategies for enhancing each type of intelligence and invites participants to note strategies they find intriguing by Hi-lighting the activity on the worksheet, or adding it to the list.

● **Verbal/linguistic intelligence** is awakened by the spoken word; by reading someone's ideas or poetry; and by writing one's own ideas, thoughts, or poetry. To activate this intelligence: read a story and write your own sequel; engage in discussion; expand your vocabulary by learning a new word each day and using it; make a speech on an intriguing topic; or keep a journal or log.

● **Logical/mathematical intelligence** is activated in situations requiring problem solving or meeting a new challenge. To activate this intelligence: outline an issue; practice analytical thinking by comparing and contrasting; create a convincing, rational explanation for something that is totally absurd; or participate in a project requiring use of "scientific method," such as following a recipe.

● The key sensory base of **visual/spatial intelligence** is the sense of sight, but also the ability to form images and pictures in the mind. To catalyze your visual/spatial intelligence: work with "artistic media" to express an idea or opinion; do intentional daydreaming; practice internal exercises such as visualizing a problem as a construction project; or use various design skills such as drawing diagrams to convey your ideas.

- Our bodies are very wise. They know things our minds don't and can't know in any other way. To call your **body/kinesthetic intelligence** to the fore: act out an idea; opinion, or feeling; play noncompetitive games and practice activities that require lots of movement; or carefully observe yourself involved in everyday tasks to become aware of what your body knows and how it functions.

- Of all forms of intelligence the *consciousness altering* effect of music and rhythm on the brain is the greatest. To activate your **musical/ rhythmic knowing**: listen to different kinds of music to shift your mood; use singing to express an idea; hum to create different kinds of vibrations inside of your head; or ask yourself what you can learn from the rhythms and patterns of nature.

- **Interpersonal intelligence** is usually essential for nurturing relationships at home, and working productively with others on the job. To awaken this intelligence: get involved in a committee or team; practice listening deeply and fully to another person; pay attention to various nonverbal cues, then check your accuracy of perception; or explore different ways to communicate with someone else.

- Our self-identity and the ability to transcend the self are part of the functioning of **intrapersonal intelligence**. According to Gardner, this intelligence is the most private and requires all other intelligence forms to express itself. To activate intrapersonal intelligence: periodically practice acute mindfulness (intense awareness of everything going on); watch your thoughts, feelings, and moods as if you were a detached, outside observer; and objectify your various thinking strategies and patterns; or answer the question "Who am I?" in 25 words or less.

VARIATIONS

- To simplify the process, combine *Steps 8, 14,* and *15* as part of the process in *Step 6*.

- Feel free to substitute other content for the group activities in *Step 11*. Participants could design their projects on self-care techniques, stress management, fitness, or any topic that fits the goals of your teaching.

*This exercise is based on the work of Dr. David Lazear, author of the mind-boggling book **Seven Ways of Knowing** (Palatine IL:IRI/Skylight Publishing, 1991). Everyone who teaches adults or children in any setting should take this book to heart.*

SEVEN WAYS OF KNOWING WORKSHEET

TYPE/ QUALITIES	CAPACITIES	ACTIVITIES
Verbal/ Linguistic	Understanding the order and meaning of words Convincing someone of a course of action Explaining, teaching, and learning Humor Memory and recall "Meta-linguistic" analysis	◆ Reading ◆ Vocabulary ◆ Formal speech ◆ Creative writing ◆ Poetry ◆ Verbal debate ◆ Impromptu speaking ◆ Humor/jokes ◆ Storytelling ◆ Journal/diary keeping
Logical/ Mathematical	Abstract pattern recognition Inductive reasoning Deductive reasoning Discerning relationships and connections Performing complex calculations Scientific reasoning	◆ Abstract symbols/formulas ◆ Out-lining ◆ Graphic organizers ◆ Number sequences ◆ Calculation ◆ Deciphering codes ◆ Forcing relationships ◆ Syllogisms ◆ Problem solving ◆ Pattern games
Visual/ Spatial	Accurate perception from different angles Recognizing relationships of objects in space Graphic representation Image manipulation Finding your way in space Forming mental images Active imagination	◆ Guided imagery ◆ Active imagination ◆ Color schemes ◆ Patterns/designs ◆ Painting ◆ Drawing mind-mapping ◆ Pretending ◆ Sculpture ◆ Pictures
Body/ Kinesthetic	Control of voluntary movements Control of "pre-programed" movements Expanding awareness through the body Mind/body connection Mimetic abilities Improved body functions	◆ Folk/creative dance ◆ Role playing ◆ Physical gestures ◆ Drama ◆ Martial arts ◆ Body language ◆ Physical exercise ◆ Mime ◆ Inventing ◆ Sports games
Musical/ Rhythmic	Structure of music "Schemas" for hearing music Sensitivity to sounds Creating melody/rhythm Sensing qualities of a tone	◆ Rhythmic patterns ◆ Vocal sounds ◆ Music composition/creation ◆ Percussion vibrations ◆ Humming ◆ Environmental sounds ◆ Singing ◆ Instrumental sounds ◆ Tonal patterns ◆ Music performance
Interpersonal	Creating and maintaining synergy "Passing over" into the perspective of another Working cooperatively in a group Noticing and making distinctions among others Verbal/nonverbal communications	◆ Giving/receiving feedback ◆ Intuiting feelings ◆ Cooperative learning strategies ◆ Person-to-person communication ◆ Empathy practices ◆ Collaboration ◆ Division of labor ◆ Sensing others' motives ◆ Group projects
Intrapersonal	Concentration of the mind Mindfulness Metacognition Awareness and expression of different feelings Transpersonal sense of the self Higher order thinking/reasoning	◆ Silent reflection methods ◆ Thinking strategies ◆ Emotional processing ◆ "Know thyself" procedures ◆ Mind-fulness/centering practices ◆ Focusing/concentration skills ◆ Higher-order reasoning ◆ Complex guided imagery

163 RELATIONSHIP REPORT CARD

Participants examine the health of their primary relationships and friendships by completing a report card covering positive and negative characteristics for each relationship.

GOALS

To promote healthy relationships.

To reflect on which relationships to nurture, which to release, and where to
build new relationships.

GROUP SIZE

Unlimited. This exercise is easily adapted for use with individuals.

TIME FRAME

30–40 minutes

MATERIALS NEEDED

One copy of the **Relationship Report Card** worksheet for each participant;
sheets of newsprint and markers for each small group; masking tape.

PROCESS

1) The trainer provides an introductory chalktalk about the importance of
   healthy relationships for personal well-being.

   ● **Healthy relationships help keep you well.** Indigenous people and
     Eastern cultures have known this for centuries. Our ancestors recog-
     nized that interdependence is necessary for survival. Individuals who
     are alienated or cut off from their family, community, or tribe are at
     higher risk for illness or death. Those who have strong, meaningful,
     loving connections to others live longer, are more resistant to stress
     and illness, and enjoy more satisfying lives.

   ● **Healthy relationships are balanced by give and take** where efforts
     are made to satisfy the needs of both people. Mutual respect leads to
     a rich exchange of resources: time, energy, affection, support,
     material possessions, knowledge, skills, intimacy, cultural traditions,
     and much more. This sharing promotes the personal growth of each
     person and leaves each richer in self-respect and self-esteem.

©1995 Whole Person Press 210 W Michigan Duluth MN 55802   (800) 247-6789

● **To stay healthy, we need more than one relationship.** No one person can meet all our needs and expectations. We need a rich variety of relationships which can meet our complex needs for growth, challenge, intimacy, nurturing, achievement, play, regeneration, work, and companionship.

2) The trainer distributes copies of the **Relationship Report Card** worksheet to each participant, and challenges them to reflect on the health of their current relationships.

➤ Write names of your same sex friends, opposite sex friends, and primary relationships (past and present) in the space provided at the top of the **Report Card**.

➤ Take a minute to consider each relationship in the light of **how that person behaves** toward you.

➢ In the boxes under each person's name, put a small ✗ opposite any of the positive or negative characteristics that person displays toward you in your relationship.

➢ Take time to consider each relationship and how you feel about it.

➢ Jot down notes to yourself on the margins of your worksheet.

   ☞ *Pause 3–5 minutes, or until most people seem to be finished.*

➤ Now look at the larger picture of the three groups (same and opposite sex friends and primary/family relationships).

➢ Are they balanced?

➢ Note your observations.

   ☞ *Pause briefly.*

➤ Now consider how you behave in each of these relationships.

➢ In the boxes under each person's name, put an ○ opposite any of the positive or negative characteristics that **you display** to them in your relationship. (Some boxes will be empty, some will have either an ✗ or ○, and some will have both.)

➢ Again, consider each relationship and how you feel about it.

➢ Jot notes as needed.

   ☞ *Pause 3–5 minutes.*

➢ Now look at the three groupings again and decide if they're balanced for you.

➢ Write notes to yourself about your observations.

   ☞ *Pause briefly.*

➤ Finally, look over your **Report Card** and make some resolutions about your relationships. Which ones need nurturing? Which ones should you release? Where do you need or want to build relationships?

3) The trainer instructs participants to form small groups of 4–6 people according to their interest in **nuturing**, **releasing**, or **building** relationships. He passes our a sheet of newsprint and marker to each small group, and gives instructions for group sharing.

➤ Each person take 2 minutes to share anything you want about your **Relationship Report Card**.

➤ The person with the biggest watch is appointed timekeeper.

☞ *Interrupt after 8–10 minutes and remind groups of their themes.*

➤ Now take 4 minutes to brainstorm, as a group, strategies for your chosen group theme: how to nurture, release, or build new relationships.

➤ The person with the shortest writing utensil is recorder.

➤ Write your theme on the top of your newsprint.

➤ Record all ideas on your newsprint.

4) The trainer invites group reporters to present their ideas to the large group.

☞ *Summarize as ideas are presented and post the lists.*

5) The trainer concludes by challenging participants to nourish themselves with rich, healthy relationships, and offers practical tips for doing so.

● **Give yourself periodic relationship checkups.** Chances are you undergo physical checkups to maintain body wellness. Why not do the same for your relationships? Take time to reflect, analyze your feelings, and decide what is needed. You may have outgrown some relationships, and need to move on. Others may be bad for you, and need ending. Some may need an injection of variety or other life spices.

● **Think of a relationship as a third person or system** that is bigger than you and the other person. It has a life of its own. What does it need to grow and stay alive?

● **Value relationship investments.** Put time, energy, and commitment into healthy relationships. These deposits will yield rich returns in the short and long run: better health and happiness.

Submitted by Krysta Kavenaugh.

RELATIONSHIP REPORT CARD

Characteristics	Same Sex Friends						Opposite Sex Friends						Primary Relationships (past and present)					
Names																		
POSITIVE																		
Common interests																		
Good communication																		
Nurturing																		
Accepting																		
Trustworthy																		
Loyal																		
Fun to be with																		
Romantic																		
Good sex																		
Right amount of time together																		
Open, sharing, supportive																		
Appreciates you																		
Respects your privacy																		
Shares responsibilities																		
Resolves conflicts fairly																		
NEGATIVE																		
Demanding																		
Critical																		
Distant																		
Manipulative																		
Boring																		
Tries to change you																		
You can't be you																		
Undependable																		
Violent																		
Overly dependent																		
Dishonest																		
Avoids/mishandles conflict																		
Violates your privacy																		

164 SPIRITUAL FINGERPRINT

In this playful, right-brain exercise, participants create an art work which symbolizes their current spirituality and then reflect upon ways to nourish their spirit.

GOALS

To explore personal spirituality from a new perspective.

To identify spiritual needs and ways to nurture them.

GROUP SIZE

Unlimited.

TIME FRAME

60 minutes

MATERIALS NEEDED

Drawing paper or large sheets of construction paper, crayons, colored markers, water colors, fingerpaints, clay, yarn, magazines, glue, scissors, and other miscellaneous art and craft supplies for each participant. Also include a blank paper for each person and large newsprint for the trainer.

PROCESS

1) The trainer distributes small, blank sheets of paper to each participant and invites group members to write down their own definition of spirituality.

2) The trainer directs participants to pair up with a neighbor and read their definitions, briefly explaining the reason they chose this definition.

3) When participants have finished sharing their definitions, the trainer suggests that there are probably as many different definitions of spirituality as there are different people in the group.

   ● Our personal spirituality is as distinctive as our fingerprints. Diversity affirms our uniqueness. Each person's definition is right for them. It is important for all to respect and accept the different beliefs of everyone present.

4) Participants are advised to put their definitions of spirituality in their pocket, purse, or wallet, and save it for reference later in the exercise. The trainer continues with a broad definition of spirituality.

● **Spirituality refers to the flow of life.** The word spirit comes from the Latin word *spiritus*, which means breath of life. When we talk about spirituality, we are describing a flow of energy that moves through us and affects our movements, our attitudes, our feelings, and our connections with other people.

● **Spirituality is different from religion.** Religion is the service or adoration of God, or a god, as expressed in doctrines and forms of worship. Spirituality cuts across all religious traditions, and involves the essence of what gives us life and meaning.

● **Your current spirituality is a composite of many forces**: your personal history, religious and philosophical traditions, joyful and painful experiences, relationships with others, belief in a higher power, and overall health and wellness.

5) The trainer coaches participants to think about the kinds of things affecting their current spirituality and asks a series of questions to prompt exploration.

☞ *Create your own examples or use those provided to stimulate thinking about each question.*

✔ What are some of your current joys and disappointments? (eg, new grandchildren, death of a friend)

✔ How would you symbolize these? (eg, Alpha and Omega)

✔ How does your work provide meaning for you? (eg, altruism, painful challenge)

✔ What aspects of your intimate relationships shape your spirituality? (eg, love and trust, betrayal)

✔ How does your current family impact your spirituality? (eg, inspiration)

✔ What old pattern or themes keep popping up in the present? (eg, overwork, faith in times of crisis)

6) The trainer announces that group members will now create an art form to represent their spiritual fingerprint, reminding participants that no two will be alike, because everyone is unique.

☞ *Move the table of art supplies to a central location and explain the process.*

➤ Feel free to get up and move to a comfortable place of the room to do your fingerprint.

➢ It is okay to sit on the floor if you choose.

➤ Use any of the art supplies provided to create your spiritual finger-print.

➤ You may draw, write, paint, cut and paste, or sculpt your spiritu-ality in any way that has meaning for you.

➤ You will have 30 minutes to complete your fingerprint.

➤ Do not think too hard about this project. Allow yourself to become spontaneous and rely on your intuition.

➤ If you want, work with your opposite hand to free the child within and access your deepest emotions.

☞ *Announce when time is half up, then remind participants when they have 5 minutes left to complete their project.*

7) When everyone has finished their fingerprint, the trainer asks partici-pants to find their original partner. When everyone has reconnected, the trainer encourages them to talk about their fingerprints.

➤ Decide who is ***Confucius*** and who is ***Buddha***.

➤ Each person should take 5 minutes to tell the story behind your spiritual fingerprint.

➤ When one person is talking, the other should listen attentively and refrain from interrupting. Accept your partner's spiritual finger-print without judgment.

➤ ***Buddhas*** begin and continue describing your fingerprints until time is called.

☞ *Inform the group when 5 minutes have passed, and instruct them to reverse roles so* ***Confucius*** *can talk.*

8) When most pairs are finished sharing, the trainer distributes blank paper and challenges participants to take a few minutes to reflect on the meaning of their fingerprints.

➤ What questions surfaced for you in this process?

➤ What truths emerged?

➤ What actions are needed to challenge and nurture you spirituality?

9) After participants have had time to reflect and record insights, the trainer directs them to take out their definition of spirituality written at the beginning of the session.

➤ Read your definition again.

➤ Does your definition of spirituality fit with the artistic rendering of your spiritual fingerprint?

➤ Would you like to modify your definition of spirituality in any way?

➤ If so, write your new definition on the sheet with your first definition.

10) The trainer concludes with a chalktalk encouraging participants to care for their spirituality as they would their minds, bodies, and relationships.

● **Pay attention to what has heart and meaning for you and nourish your life force.** If the sound of water soothes your soul, spend time by the lake or ocean—or listen to audiotapes of the ocean or a babbling brook. If prayer and meditation help you achieve peace of mind, set aside quiet time for yourself. If helping others is central to your spirituality, volunteer at a hospital or church. If nature makes you feel close to God, spend time outdoors. By listening to your spirit and responding with care, you'll enrich your life and develop a deeper sense of well-being.

● **Develop traditions, rituals, and ceremonies** that nourish your spirit. Evening prayers or poems, daily expressions of love and gratitude, seasonal challenges to do something you've never done before, letters of apology or forgiveness, dancing, singing, listening to music are all possible rituals you could incorporate into your life. These ceremonies will reinforce the values that are most important to you.

11) The trainer ends the learning session by recommending that participants hang or display their spiritual fingerprints somewhere in their home, pointing out that this will be a visual reminder of their life force, and the importance of nuturing their spirituality.

VARIATIONS

■ Participants hang or display their spiritual fingerprints around the room, and then tour the "gallery" and talk with people about the meaning of their symbols.

Submitted by John Sippola.

165 LEISURE PURSUITS

In this expansive assessment and exploration of the needs met by work and play, participants discover their priorities and possibilities for leisure pursuits.

GOALS

To evaluate the balance between work and leisure.

To identify needs met by work and leisure pursuits.

To explore affirmative activities for meeting leisure needs.

GROUP SIZE

Unlimited.

TIME FRAME

20–30 minutes

MATERIALS NEEDED

Pie Chart (p 36) and **Leisure Pursuits** worksheets for all; newsprint or marker board.

PROCESS

☞ *This exercise uses a worksheet from Pie Charts, p 36.*

1) The trainer distributes **Pie Charts** worksheets and invites participants to consider the balance between work and leisure in their lives, using a pie chart.

   ➤ Imagine this pie represents your time and energy.

     ➢ Divide the pie into two sections that represent the amount of time and energy you spend **working** (including working around the house as well as paid work and volunteer work), and the amount of time and energy you spend at **leisure**.

     ➢ Label the sections appropriately.

   ➤ Now consider what **personal needs** of yours are met by these two different dimensions of life.

     ➢ Jot down in the **work segment** of your pie some of the satisfactions you gain from your work wherever it is, some of the needs it meets for you.

➤ In the **leisure segment** of your pie, write down the activities you typically engage in during your leisure time and note what needs are met and what satisfactions you receive. Don't forget about sex and cat napping!

➤ Make a comment on the bottom of your worksheet indicating how you feel about your current balance and what changes you might consider making.

2) Participants pair up and compare pie charts. (2–3 minutes)

3) The trainer reconvenes the group and solicits examples of what participants do in their leisure time, and transforms these contributions into statements of **underlying needs**.

☞ Rephrase each response, asking the participant, "What are you looking for with this activity? What are you seeking or pursuing?"

4) As the group offers examples of leisure pursuits, the trainer compiles a list of **needs** on the newsprint or marker board.

☞ You may need to challenge the group to think more creatively about possible leisure needs: competition, helping, self awareness,, relaxation, interaction, physical release, risk taking, pride in accomplishments, personal space, adventure, power, fun, creativity, spiritual renewal, etc. The more comprehensive (and imaginative) the list, the better.

5) The trainer distributes the **Leisure Pursuits** worksheets and notes that sometimes we get the same type of rewards from work and leisure, but for most of us, variety would be better.

➤ Focus on the **work portion** of your pie again, considering your needs that are typically met by your work.

➤ On the **top** of your **Leisure Pursuits** worksheet, complete the sentence stems about your work.

6) When most people have identified their work needs, the trainer invites them to focus on their leisure pursuits.

➤ Given where your are in your life right now, what needs would you like to meet through your leisure activities?

➤ On the **bottom half** of the worksheet, list eight or ten things you **need from your leisure time** these days.

☞ Remind folks to search the lists you generated earlier for relevant needs.

7) When all have made their lists the trainer instructs participants to rank these needs in order, with 1 being the most important need, down to 8 or 10 as least important.

8) When the rankings are complete, the trainer asks partners from *Step 2* to join another pair to make quartets and gives instructions for sharing and brainstorming.

> ➤ Each person will state the top-priority need you would like to satisfy during leisure time and what activity you would typically choose to meet that need.
>
> > ➤ Take turns.
> >
> > ➤ The person with the most years of working fulltime goes first.
>
> ➤ The other three group members will then brainstorm all the additional leisure pursuits they can imagine would meet this need for you.
>
> > ➤ Take notes on intriguing possibilities suggested by the group.
>
> ➤ When the creative energy peters out, move to the next person on the right, and repeat the process with that person's top-priority need.
>
> ➤ If you get all the way around the group before time is called, start over again, using your number two priority needs.
>
> ☞ *Wander around and make sure all groups have made at least one complete loop before moving on to the next step.*

9) The trainer interrupts and directs participants to look over the leisure pursuits they have listed during this process and make a **personal resolution about leisure** to write at the bottom of their worksheet.

10) The trainer reconvenes the larger group and asks each person to read her resolution out loud, then closes the session with a resolution of her own.

LEISURE PURSUITS WORKSHEET

My work gives me . . .

_____   _____
_____   _____
_____   _____
_____   _____
_____   _____
_____   _____
_____   _____

In my leisure time I need . . .   Group ideas:

_____
_____
_____
_____
_____
_____
_____
_____
_____
_____
_____

Resolution:

Planning
& Closure

166 COMMERCIAL SUCCESS

This exercise provides a creative way for participants to synthesize learning at the end of a session, working in teams to develop and perform a commercial to sell key ideas to the public.

GOALS

To summarize information and reinforce learning.

To be creative and have fun.

GROUP SIZE

Works best for groups of 15-30 people.

TIME FRAME

15–20 minutes

PROCESS

1) The trainer announces that he has just been contacted by a Madison Avenue ad agency that needs some actors to perform in a commercial. The trainer then says, "Guess what, you are the actors."

   ☞ *Inevitably you will hear groans from the group as people react to the idea of having to perform. Respond by saying, "I heard a few groans, but they were not good enough. I'll bet you can groan better than that. Let's try again. I'll count to three and you groan as loud as you can. . .1, 2, 3, groan." Then say "Great! You are obviously the talented actors we need. Now, let's get to work."*

2) The trainer instructs participants to return to small groups from earlier in the session and challenges them to integrate their learning by developing a commercial to sell their ideas to the public.

   ➤ Develop a 60-second commercial advertising one or more key ideas and concepts from the learning session.

      ➢ The commercial needs to persuade the public why the content of the session was important, and how they will benefit from it.

   ➤ You have 10 minutes to develop the commercial and then perform your commercial for the large group.

      ➢ Have fun and be creative.

➤ Include everyone in your group as part of the commercial.

☞ *Remind people when time is half up, and again when there is one minute left until showtime.*

3) The trainer invites each group to come to the front of the room and perform their commercial.

☞ *Lead the group in enthusiastic applause for each group when they finish their commercial performance.*

4) The facilitator invites participants to discuss the process of developing their commercial using several questions.

✔ What was the hardest part of this exercise?

✔ What part did you enjoy the most?

✔ How do you think working as a team affected the quality of your commercial?

5) The trainer weaves group responses in a chalktalk summarizing the learning process.

● When you synthesize learning, you are more likely to remember it. By creating a commercial, you reinforced ideas important to you, which will help you with ongoing decisions about your health.

● Remember to continue to sell yourself on wellness and take an active role in promoting it for yourself and others.

TRAINER'S NOTES

Submitted by Mark Warner.

167 IF . . . THEN

This quick and easy planner challenges participants to imagine the consequences of continuing or changing their present health-related behaviors.

GOALS

To review insights learned about wellness.

To apply learning by planning for positive behavioral changes.

GROUP SIZE

Unlimited.

TIME FRAME

15–20 minutes

MATERIALS NEEDED

One copy of the **If . . .Then** worksheet for each participant, large newsprint
and marker.

PROCESS

1) The trainer draws a large box on newsprint, and divides it in half
   vertically by drawing a line down the middle, creating two columns.
   She writes **If I continue . . .** on the top of the left column, and writes
   Then . . . on the top of the right column.

2) The trainer then invites participants to consider the consequences of
   health-related behaviors.

   ✔ What are some examples of behaviors that will positively or nega-
   tively affect a person's health if they are continued?

   ☞ *Give several examples from earlier in the session. (Eg, "If I*
   continue to work through my lunch hour, I might suffer burn-
   out." "If I continue daily walks, I will become more fit and lose
   weight.")

3) As participants brainstorm behaviors and consequences/outcomes, the
   trainer records them in the **If . . .** and **Then . . .** sections of the newsprint.

   ☞ *Prod the group to consider health-related behaviors that affect*
   their work, their personal relationships, their physical health, their
   mental outlook, and other categories relevant to the group.

4) The trainer observes that just as negative health habits can lead to unpleasant consequences, positive changes can lead to improved health. She announces that participants will now focus on one health-related behavior that they want to change.

5) The trainer distributes **If . . . Then** worksheets and invites participants to reflect on behaviors they want to change.

➤ Focus on a specific health-related behavior you need and want to change because of its negative effect on your well-being (physical, mental, or spiritual).

➢ In the top box of the worksheet, after the words **If I continue . . .** write the particular behavior that you want to **change**.

➢ After the word **Then . . .** write all the possible consequences of **continuing** your present behavior.

➤ Now think of a more positive behavior you want to substitute for the old one.

➢ Write a description of this health-enhancing behavior in the section labeled **Instead, if I . . .**

➢ In the bottom section, after the word, **Then . . .** write down all the possible consequences or outcomes of engaging in this new behavior.

➤ Look over your worksheet and put a star beside any consequences or outcomes you think are positive.

6) When nearly everyone is finished, the trainer instructs participants to return to their original small group and share their worksheet.

➤ Each person has about one minute to share what you have written on your worksheet.

7) The trainer ends the small group discussions and advises participants to remember the **If . . . Then** principle and use it as a guide for making healthy choices about their health.

VARIATIONS

■ Instead of using a worksheet for this planning process, participants complete sentences verbally in a small group round-robin. Other group members may add to each person's list of positive and negative consequences.

For a closing affirmation, ask participants to declare a commitment to changing a behavior, completing a second sentence: **I will . . . and then . . .**

IF . . . THEN

IF *I continue . . .*

Then...

INSTEAD

If *I . . .*

Then...

168 JUST FOR TODAY

This memorable planning process based on the twelve steps challenges participants to make concrete commitments to change.

GOALS

To identify specific short term goals to improve well-being.

To renew commitment to change.

GROUP SIZE

Unlimited.

TIME FRAME

15–20 minutes

MATERIALS NEEDED

Just for Today worksheets for all participants.

PROCESS

1) The trainer begins with a brief chalktalk on the dynamics of change, and the role of personal resolutions.

   ● Most of us have agendas for change that are overwhelming, and often unrealistic .

   ● The best way to tackle change is one step at a time, one day at a time.

2) The trainer reads the **Just for Today** script.

   ☞ *Be sure to tell participants the source of this wisdom: Dear Abby adapted the traditional AA credo for use in her annual New Years column.*

3) The trainer distributes **Just for Today** worksheets and invites participants to reflect on how the credo applies to their current life situation and personal goals as uncovered during this learning experience..

JUST FOR TODAY Script

Just for today I will live through this day only, and not set far-reaching goals to try to overcome all my problems at once. I know I can do something for twelve hours that would appall me if I felt that I had to keep it up for a lifetime.

Just for today I will be happy. Abraham Lincoln said, "Most folks are about as happy as they make up their minds to be." He was right. I will not dwell on thoughts that depress me. I will chase them out of my mind and replace them with happy thoughts.

Just for today, I will adjust myself to what is. I will face reality. I will change those things that I can change and accept those things I cannot change.

Just for today, I will improve my mind. I will not be a mental loafer. I will force myself to read something that requires effort, thought, and concentration.

Just for today, I will do something positive to improve my health. If I'm a smoker, I'll make an honest effort to cut down. If I'm overweight, I'll eat nothing I know is fattening. And I will force myself to exercise—even if it's only walking around the block or using the stairs instead of the elevator.

Just for today, I will be totally honest. If someone asks me something I don't know, I will not bluff: I'll simply say, "I don't know."

Just for today, I'll do something I've been putting off for a long time. I'll finally write that letter, make that phone call, clean that closet, or straighten out those dresser drawers.

Just for today, before I speak I will ask myself, "Is it true? Is it kind?" And if the answer to either of those questions is negative, I won't say it.

Just for today, I will make a conscious effort to be agreeable. I will look as good as I can, dress becomingly, talk softly, act courageously and not interrupt when someone else is talking.

Just for today I'll not improve anybody except myself.

Just for today, I will have a program. I may not follow it exactly, but I will have it, thereby saving myself from two pests: hurry and indecision.

Just for today, I will have a quiet half hour to relax alone. During this time I will reflect on my behavior and get a better perspective on my life.

Just for today, I will be unafraid. I will gather the courage to do what is right and take the responsibility for my own actions. I will expect nothing from the world, but I will realize that as I give to the world, the world will give to me.

JUST FOR TODAY

I WILL LIVE FOR TODAY ONLY
What difficulties do I need to "live with"?

One focus I need to keep in mind:

One habit I won't engage in today:

One opportunity I'm going to say "yes" to:

What "worries" about tomorrow do I need to save for tomorrow?

I WILL BE HAPPY
What depressing or stressful thoughts do I need to banish?

What happy thoughts can replace them?

Ten things I can be happy about:

I WILL ADJUST MYSELF TO REALITY
What things in my life can I change?

What things can't be changed? What do I need to accept as is?

I WILL IMPROVE MY MIND
What can I do today to improve my mind?

What will I read? (newspaper, book, magazine)

Who has good ideas I can learn from today?

Perhaps someone in this class?

I WILL IMPROVE MY HEALTH
What can I do today to improve my health? (nutrition, exercise, cigarettes, alcohol, self-care routines, preventive action)

I WILL BE TOTALLY HONEST

When am I likely to fib my way through an uncomfortable situation?

With whom will I need to be especially careful to be honest?

I'LL DO SOMETHING I'VE BEEN PUTTING OFF

Where have I been procrastinating or avoiding taking action?
List several and then choose one for a focus tomorrow.

BEFORE I SPEAK I WILL ASK MYSELF, "IS IT TRUE? IS IT KIND?"

Where will I especially need to be truthful and kind in what I say?

I WILL MAKE A CONSCIOUS EFFORT TO BE AGREEABLE

What can I do to clean up my act?

When will I need to be particularly focused on being patient and courteous?

I'LL NOT IMPROVE ANYBODY ELSE BUT MYSELF

When am I most tempted to criticize others?

Where am I likely to pass judgment on another rather than myself?

I'LL HAVE A PROGRAM

What am I trying to accomplish with my day?

What clear behaviors and attitudes will I focus on for today?

I WILL HAVE A QUIET HALF-HOUR TO RELAX ALONE

When will I take my half-hour relaxation break today?

How will I spend that time?

I WILL BE UNAFRAID

What am I most anxious about?

Where will I particularly need courage?

What can I do to conquer my fear or anxiety?

169 SELF-CARE BOUQUET

In this unique process for planning and closure, participants create a meta-phorical mixture of flower essences designed to heal their hearts, minds, and spirits.

GOALS

To identify and affirm self-care needs.

To integrate learning about wellness.

To provide closure.

GROUP SIZE

Unlimited.

TIME FRAME

20–30 minutes

MATERIALS NEEDED

One copy of the **Garden of Remedies** handout and a sheet of blank paper and crayons or colored markers for each participant.

PROCESS

1) The trainer introduces Bach's flower remedies as a metaphor for the natural approach to self-care.

- Dr. Edward Bach (1886–1936), researcher, physician, and healer, believed that the ills of the heart and spirit must be the focus of a healer's attention. Using homeopathic principles and 38 non-poison-ous plants he developed herbal remedies to restore inner harmony and balance. Dr. Bach's remedies have no scientific explanation, but there are thousands of successful case histories where these remedies were effective in restoring calm, hope, confidence, patience, and peace of mind.

- Bach's system can serve as a metaphor for us, as we activate our own healing energies toward a healthier lifestyle and self-care actions for restoring and maintaining harmony and balance in body, mind, and spirit.

- Wellness is associated with loving, positive, grateful, and forgiving attitudes and outlooks. By paying attention to how we are living and loving, we can identify simple, natural ways of healing. We can care for ourselves by attending to our inner struggles and conflicts, and thinking about what we need to do in order to develop or maintain a state of congruence, calm, and positive connection to others.

2) The trainer distributes **Garden of Remedies** worksheets and describes how to use it as a metaphor for self-care.

- ● Bach's 38 remedies are organized into seven categories that are symptoms of being out of harmony or balance: Fear, Uncertainty, Lack of Interest in the Present, Loneliness, Over-sensitivity to the Influence of Others, Despondency or Despair, and Over-Care of Others. Most of us can identify with one or more of these.

- ● Bach discovered a 39th remedy for real emergencies. The rescue remedy is used in times of severe trauma and stress. It includes Rock Rose for terror or panic, Cherry Plum to help a person stay in control when they are hysterical, Impatiens for calming down, Clematis for clear thinking in an emergency, and Star of Bethlehem for neutralizing trauma or fright. Most of us have also experienced like situations where we needed such a remedy.

- ➤ Look over Bach's list of symptoms again and think about the self-care you need at this time in your life.

  - ➣ Circle 4–6 flower remedies that sound like they might represent the healing you need in your current struggles and conflicts.

3) The trainer distributes blank paper and crayons or markers, and invites participants to make a self-care bouquet.

- ➤ Draw a self-care bouquet using your chosen flower remedies.

  - ➣ Don't worry about artistic skills or accuracy.

  - ➣ Represent the flower remedies in any way you want. Arrange them in any combination, color or design.

  - ➣ Add any other self-care remedies you might need that weren't on the list, and give them a fanciful botanical name.

  - ➣ Create your own personalized vessel to hold the flowers.

4) When participants have finished their self-care bouquets, the trainer asks group members to return to their small groups for sharing and planning.

- ➤ Select one person to be timekeeper.

- ➤ Each person has two minutes to show the group your bouquet, tell about the remedies you have selected, and explain why they were chosen.

5) After 8–10 minutes, when everyone has described their bouquets, the trainer describes the next step.

➤ Think about what you need to do to apply these self-care remedies to your current life.

➤ Jot down three ideas for what you will do to make these remedies a reality.

➤ Go around the group again, and share your applications with each other.

6) The trainer reconvenes the group and asks for testimonials or other closing insights.

☞ *Make a self-care bouquet from you to the group. Use it to reinforce concepts and provide a closing affirmation.*

VARIATIONS

■ Group members make bouquets for each other and explain their choices.

■ Participants interested in learning about the actual Bach Flower Essences and Remedies can find books and other information at health food stores, or holistic/new age bookshops.

TRAINER'S NOTES

For more information on Bach flower remedies, check out **The Bach Flower Remedies** *by Edward Bach, MD, and F.J. Wheeler, MD (New Canaan CT: Keats Publishing Inc, 1977) which we used for developing the list of self-care options in this exercise.*

GARDEN REMEDIES

Fear

ROCK ROSE—rescue remedy for sudden illness, accident

MIMULUS—fear of everyday life and misfortune (illness, pain, control, accidents, being alone)

CHERRY PLUM—fear of loss of control of the mind or impulses, desperate

ASPEN—vague anxiety, dread

RED CHESTNUT—anxiety and worry about others

Lack of Interest in the Present

CLEMATIS—dreamy, living more in the future than the present

HONEYSUCKLE—living in the past

WILD ROSE—resigned, bored and apathetic about life

OLIVE—mental and physical exhaustion

WHITE CHESTNUT—worry, unpleasant thoughts

MUSTARD—gloom and despair

CHESTNUT BUD—repeat mistakes and same difficulties

Over-Sensitivity to Influence of Others

AGRONOMY—peacemakers who avoid conflict, hide their feeling with humor

CENTAURY—over-anxious to please, try too hard, overwork

WALNUT—led away from own ideas by opinions of others

HOLLY—jealousy, envy, revenge, suspicion

Over-Care for Others

BEECH—overly critical on self and others

ROCK WATER—those who are strict, hard masters to themselves

CHICORY—over-full of care of children, family, and friends; martyrs

VERVAIN—fixed principles and ideas, strong will and courage, hard-working and intense

VINE—capable, confident people who enjoy power, dominate others

Uncertainty

CERATO—lack of confidence in one's ability to make decisions

SCLERANTHUS—unable to decide between two things

GENTIAN—easily discouraged

GORSE—hopelessness

HORNBEEM—feeling a lack of mental or physical strength to face life scenes

WILD OAT—strong ambitions but difficulty deciding upon a life occupation

OAK—brave people fighting against difficulty, without loss of hope

CRAB APPLE—remedy of cleansing mental and physical wounds

Loneliness

WATER VIOLET—quiet, independent, aloof, peaceful people who like to be alone

IMPATIENS—impatient with themselves and others, irritable

HEATHER—dependent on others, unhappy alone, obsessed with own problems

Despondency or Despair

LARCH—low self-esteem or self-worth, lack of self-confidence

PINE—guilt and self-blame

ELM—talented achievers or humanitarians who suffer bouts of depression and uncertainty, feel overwhelmed

SWEET CHESTNUT—unbearable anguish

STAR OF BETHLEHEM—great distress, shock, loss, and trauma

WILLOW—bitterness resulting from adversity or misfortune

39th Combination Remedy for Rescue

CLEMATIS—for clear thinking in an emergency

IMPATIENS—for pain, impatience, nervousness that accompanies severe stress

ROCK ROSE—for terror, panic

CHERRY PLUM—desperation, fear of loss of control at time of shock

STAR OF BETHLEHEM—for neutralizing the effects of trauma

170 TAKE THE PLEDGE

The power of a promise is apparent in this light-hearted closing pledge of allegiance to wellness goals.

GOALS

To make a commitment to personal health goals.

To experience closure for group process.

GROUP SIZE

Unlimited.

TIME FRAME

10–15 minutes

MATERIALS NEEDED

Taking the Pledge worksheets.

PROCESS

1) The trainer suggests that participants rejoin their small group for this closing exercise. Once groups are settled, she invites everyone to choose a goal.

   ➤ Think back over this meeting and recall the important concepts and issues about wellness that we have covered.

   ➤ Consider how you might apply these ideas to your current life.

   ➤ Decide on a health or wellness goal, that you want to achieve in the coming month or year.

2) As participants are deliberating, the trainer distributes **Taking the Pledge** worksheets, and when all have a goal in mind, she gives the next instructions.

   ➤ Okay. Now it's commitment time. Rewrite your goal in the form of a pledge of allegiance, modeled after the Pledge of Allegiance to the U.S. flag

   ☞ *Give a couple of examples (eg, I pledge allegiance to stop smoking and to the self-control for which it stands, healthy lungs, fresh air, with fresh breath and extra cash for my family).*

➤ What change are you going to make? Write it on *Line 1*.

➤ What is the value or purpose that underlies your goal? (*Line 2*)

➤ What positive outcomes do you anticipate if you reach this goal? (*Lines 3 and 4*)

➤ What additional benefits might result from this change? (*Lines 5 and 6*)

➤ Who will be affected or how long will these benefits last? (*Line 7*)

3) When everyone has written their pledge, the trainer gives instructions for sharing pledges with the group.

➤ Stand up in a circle. Each person take a turn. Put your hand on your heart and read your pledge aloud to your group.

4) The trainer concludes by suggesting that group members keep their pledges in their wallet, on the refrigerator, or in another prominent place where they can read it often and remind themselves of their goal.

VARIATIONS

■ The pledge can be applied to specialized goals, such as self-care, physical fitness, recovery and healing, self-esteem, relaxation, anger management, nutrition, etc.

■ For a humorous variation, make up tongue-in-cheek pledges. Eg, "I pledge allegiance to Staying Stressed, and to the Lifestyle for which it stands. One worry, after another, with Tension and Anxiety for all."

TRAINER'S NOTES

*Variation suggested by Doug Stewart, author of **Staying Stressed** (Santa Fe, New Mexico: High Mountain Press, 1994).*

TAKING THE PLEDGE

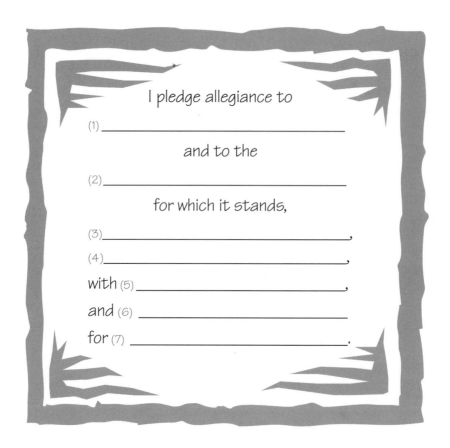

I pledge allegiance to

(1) _____

and to the

(2) _____

for which it stands,

(3) _____,

(4) _____,

with (5) _____,

and (6) _____

for (7) _____.

Group Energizers

171 CHOOSE WELLNESS ANYWAY

This lively exercise engages participants in a high-spirited litany asserting principles of wellness.

GOALS

To affirm a wellness way of life.

TIME FRAME

5–10 minutes

MATERIALS NEEDED

One copy of the **Choose Wellness Anyway** litany for each participant.

PROCESS

1) The trainer acknowledges the ongoing efforts of group members to stay well, sometimes without much support or encouragement. He announces that in this quick exercise, they will have the opportunity to form a chorus with other members and affirm a wellness way of life.

2) The trainer distributes copies of the **Choose Wellness Anyway** litany and asks participants to stand for the responsive reading.

   ➤ My job is to pose the discouraging cultural challenges to wellness.

   ➤ Your job is to reaffirm the **wellness way** using phrases in ***bold-italics***.

     ➤ Be enthusiastic. Speak with clarity and conviction.

3) The trainer reads the **Choose Wellness Anyway** litany, encouraging participants to respond with great gusto.

4) When the litany is done, the trainer invites a round of applause and cheers from the group. He then recommends that participants consider framing their wellness litany and hanging it in their home or office, as a reminder of their commitment to wellness goals.

VARIATIONS

■ Divide the group in half. One side shouts the discouraging messages. The other side responds with encouragements for wellness.

*Submitted by Don Ardell and Julie Lusk. The litany was inspired by Sal Spalenger's **Do It Anyway.***

©1995 Whole Person Press 210 W Michigan Duluth MN 55802   (800) 247-6789

CHOOSE WELLNESS ANYWAY LITANY

We can't escape the unhealthy messages all around us.
Choose wellness anyway.

If you encourage others to live well,
they might say you're a health nut.
Encourage them anyway.

If you seek balance in your mind, body, and spirit,
people may say you are self-centered.
Balance your life anyway.

The energy you expend in pursuit of personal excellence
may be more than is really necessary.
Invest in excellence anyway.

Your accomplishments and contributions
may have little lasting impact.
Achieve and contribute anyway.

Integrity and high standards will
make life more difficult.
Be the best you can be anyway.

Finding foods that nourish can be
a lot of trouble and cost you more.
Choose good food anyway.

Learning how to love the work you do is very difficult.
Learn to love it anyway.

Life is painful and filled with tragedies.
Laugh and play anyway.

We are all mortal and in time death will prevail.
Live well anyway.

By Donald B. Ardell

172 CLEANSING BREATH

Participants experiment with a yoga breathing technique that is a powerful natural tranquilizer.

GOALS

To quiet and balance the mind and emotion.

To promote relaxation.

TIME FRAME

3–5 minutes

MATERIALS NEEDED

Cleansing Breath script.

☞ *For a more thorough introduction to Yoga and its health benefits, see* **Yoga** *(Stress 5, p 94).*

PROCESS

1) The trainer introduces the exercise with a few comments on breathing and Yoga.

   ● **The goal of Yoga is a peaceful, clear mind in a sound, healthy body.** Hatha (ha-tah) Yoga approaches this goal from the physical aspect— through body postures, breathing techniques, diet, and deep relaxation.

   ● The **Cleansing Breath**, or alternate nostril breathing, calms and balances the nervous system while promoting mental focus and relaxation. This techniques is an excellent instant natural tranquilizer.

2) The trainer guides the group through the breathing technique, using the **Cleansing Breath** script.

   ☞ *To avoid confusion during the script, you may want to demonstrate the technique, showing the proper hand position for closing alternate nostrils.*

   Participants should remove their eyeglasses for this exercise.

CLEANSING BREATH Script

Sit up very tall, allowing your spine to lengthen
and your shoulders to drop into a relaxed, but balanced posture . . .

Breathe slowly and gently through your nose . . .
feeling your chest and abdomen expanding with your breath . . .
Then empty the air very slowly out of your nose again . . .
feeling your chest and your stomach relax . . .

Keep breathing deeply and gently in through your nose . . .
down into your chest and abdomen . . .
then out through your nose . . .
relaxing your chest and stomach . . .

Continue to breathe deeply and gently . . .
while you bring your right hand up to your nose . . .
Rest the tips of your first two fingers on your forehead . . .
between your eyebrows . . .
Let your thumb rest gently on one side of your nose . . .
while your ring finger and pinky finger rest gently
against the other side of your nose. . . .

Keeping the same steady rhythm to your breathing . . .
on the next inhale,
*close your **right** nostril by pressing gently with your thumb . . .*

*Inhale through the **left** nostril . . .*
and then close off your left nostril with your ring finger . . .
Hold for a count of four.
Now release your thumb
and slowly exhale through the right nostril to a count of 8 . . .

And then inhale again through your right nostril to a count of 8 . . .
Close both nostrils and hold to a count of 4 . . .
Then release your ring finger
and exhale through your left nostril to a count of 8 . . .

> ☞ *Repeat this alternating pattern for 10 breaths, main-*
> *taining the 8–4–8 count beat and changing sides before*
> *each **exhale**.*

173 FOR THE HEALTH OF IT

Group members are invited to kick up their heels in a dance for fun and fitness.

GOALS

To enjoy the health benefits of dancing.

To stimulate interest in dance as a natural and fun way to exercise.

GROUP SIZE

Unlimited. This exercise works best with groups larger than 12 people.

TIME FRAME

5–10 minutes

MATERIALS NEEDED

Trainer's choice of dance music on tape or CD available in most music stores (Bunny Hop, Butterfly, Hokey Pokey, Polka, Chicken, or folk dance); audio equipment for playing music, and a room large enough for people to move about freely.

PROCESS

1) The trainer asks everyone to stand up and perform the following movements:

   ➤ Stand with your feet together, arms at your side.

   ➤ Squat, bending your knees slowly to a 90-degree angle, lifting your arms to shoulder height.

   ➤ Return to the starting position.

2) The trainer instructs participants to sit back down, and then asks them what they think they just did. He solicits ideas, focusing on answers relating to exercise or calisthenics.

3) He then reveals that what participants have actually done is the first step of a disco routine. He points out how dance steps and calisthenics look alike, and are both a form of exercise.

4) The trainer outlines the health benefits of dancing in a short chalktalk.

● Dancing increases muscle flexibility, develops coordination.

● Dancing burns calories. Ballroom dancing will burn 250 calories an hour; more vigorous dancing (like disco) can burn up to 500 calories and hour.

● Dancing improves the condition of heart, lungs, and circulatory systems.

● Dancing releases muscle tension and promotes relaxation.

● Dancing can be a healthful activity to enjoy with friends and family. It requires no equipment except comfortable shoes, and can be enjoyed for many years.

5) The trainer announces that participants will have the opportunity to enjoy a dance with other group members, and introduces the chosen dance.

  ☞ *Expect groans and moans from the non-dancers in the group. Reassure these people that the focus here is on fun and participation, not performance. Explain that you will teach the steps, and encourage everyone to try.*

  Advise everyone to listen to their bodies and not do anything which is painful or uncomfortable for them.

6) The trainer teaches the dance by demonstrating steps and movements, and inviting group members familiar with the dance to assist in teaching other participants.

7) When everyone is familiar with the dance, the trainer turns on the music and starts the dance.

8) When the group energy starts to flag (5–8 minutes), the trainer concludes by encouraging participants to experiment with different kinds of dances, and have fun with this enjoyable form of exercise and play.

VARIATIONS

■ Participants form small groups of 4–6 people after the dance, and discuss previous positive and negative dancing experiences which have affected their feelings about dancing. The trainer solicits examples of these experiences, then instructs the groups to discuss what is needed to create more positive experiences in dancing.

Submitted by Sally Strosahl.

174 HEALTHY SING-ALONG

Everyone will enjoy this playful song, which is fun to sing and celebrates good health.

GOALS

To laugh and play as a group.

To get energized.

TIME FRAME

3–5 minutes

MATERIALS NEEDED

One copy of the **If You're Healthy** songsheet for each participant.

PROCESS

1) The trainer passes out copies of the **If You're Healthy** songsheet to each participant, and then teaches the group how to sing the song and perform the accompanying movements.

   ☞ *Demonstrate the process and asks participants to practice a trial run of one stanza.*

2) The trainer asks everyone to stand up, spread out so they have space around them to move about freely, and then sing along in unison as she leads them through the song.

   ☞ *If people seem shy or reluctant, encourage them to sing louder or shout out the words.*

VARIATIONS

■ Divide the group into three smaller groups and have each group sing one round of the song, then all sing the last section.

■ Change the lyrics to fit your course content. Group members can make up new actions to show they are healthy: dance a jig, skip around, shout olé!, breathe and sigh, stop and pray, etc.

IF YOU'RE HEALTHY SONGSHEET

(Sung to the tune of "If You're Happy and You Know It")

If you're healthy and you know it, clap your hands.

If you're healthy and you know it, clap your hands.

If you're healthy and you know it, your life will surely show it.

If you're healthy and you know it, clap your hands.

If you're healthy and you know it, run in place.

If you're healthy and you know it, run in place.

If you're healthy and you know it, your life will surely show it.

If you're healthy and you know it, clap your hands.

If you're healthy and you know it, smile and laugh—*Ha, ha, ha.*

If you're healthy and you know it, smile and laugh—*Ha, ha, ha.*

If you're healthy and you know it, your life will surely show it.

If you're healthy and you know it, smile and laugh—*Ha, ha, ha.*

If you're healthy and you know it, do all three *(clap your hands, run in place, smile and laugh—Ha, ha, ha).*

If you're healthy and you know it, do all three *(clap your hands, run in place, smile and laugh—Ha, ha, ha).*

If you're healthy and you know it, your life will surely show it.

If you're healthy and you know it, do all three *(clap your hands, run in place, smile and laugh—Ha, ha, ha).*

175 LUDICROUS WORKSHOPS

In this hilarious exercise, group members create outrageous courses for an absurd continuing education curriculum.

GOALS

To blow off steam and get energized through humor and laughter.

GROUP SIZE

Unlimited.

TIME FRAME

15–20 minutes

MATERIALS NEEDED

One copy of the **Ludicrous Workshops** handout for each participant.

PROCESS

1) The facilitator introduces this energizer by observing that everyone present obviously values continuing education or they wouldn't be attending this training. She adds that in this session, participants will have an opportunity to create their own unique courses, tailored to their special needs and interests.

2) The facilitator asks participants to form groups of six to eight people, and when this is accomplished, passes out copies of the **Ludicrous Workshop** handouts to each participant. While the sheets are being distributed, she explains that this handout lists some of the more popular continuing education courses for the stress and wellness field.

   ☞ *You could change the language here to incorporate the interest or background of group participants. For example, these courses could be described as favorites for business managers, teachers, human service professionals, emergency room nurses, busy parents, dual career families, etc.*

3) The facilitator encourages people to look over the lists and see what is currently being offered for them.

   ☞ *Participants will inevitably start to chuckle as they read their lists, and realize that this is not a serious session.*

4) The facilitator allows time for most people to read their lists and then observes that the list has a few courses on stress management. She goes on to explain the group process for creating new courses.

> ➤ Your job is to create new courses in stress management or wellness.

> ➤ Appoint a group member to be the group recorder for all of the ideas generated.

>> ➣ Be as humorous as possible making up titles which are descriptive of the course content.

>> ➣ Be careful to avoid humor that is sarcastic, offensive, or puts down individuals or groups. Also, watch for stereotyping.

>> ➣ Develop your courses with caring and empathy, involving everyone in the fun. Go ahead and poke fun at yourself or universal human foibles.

> ➤ You have 5 minutes to complete your list.

5) When time is up, the facilitator asks each group recorder to stand up one at a time and read the course descriptions for their group.

6) After all groups have shared their course lists, the facilitator asks participants which class was the most appealing to them. The responses to this question are used to end the session on a playful note, as the facilitator encourages group members to be sure to call local colleges for information about how to register for these courses.

VARIATIONS

■ The group creates ludicrous continuing education classes for their particular occupational group, corporation, agency, or area of interest.

Workshop titles submitted by David X Swenson and Mary O'Brien Sippel.

LUDICROUS WORKSHOPS

Please check any of the following courses that might interest you for continuing education.

Self Improvement

The Basics of Self-Torture
Overcoming Peace of Mind
Creative Anxiety
The Power of Negative Thinking
You and Your Birthmark
Ego Gratification Through
    One-Upmanship
Developing a Three-Dimensional
    Worry System
Visual Aids for Hallucinations
Masochist's Non-Support Group
Brooding Material for All Occasions
Discovering Your Defects
How to Channel Your Anxiety
    into Rejection
Advanced Whining
Nasal Tones for Neutrality
Getting Your Way by Screaming
Standing Up to Your Osteopath
Avoiding Intimacy at Work
    and Home
Parenting with Bribery
Self-Pity as a Conversation Opener
Guilt without Sex

Business and Career

Career Opportunities in El Salvador
How to Profit from Your Own Body
Looters' Guide to American Cities
The Underachiever's Guide to a
    Very Small Business Opportunity
"I Made $100 in Real Estate"
Investments You Can Hide
Home Course in Scuba Diving

Health and Fitness

Team Flossing
100 Ways to Duct Tape Your Droop-
    ing Eyelids
Liposuction Your Lifelines
Shallow Breathing for Energy Conser-
    vation
Guided Imagery to Inflame Your
    Nasal Membranes
Twenty Meditations for Chronic
    Constipation
Using Solar Light to Exaggerate Facial
    Blemishes
High Fiber Sex
Suicide and Your Health
Biofeedback and How to Stop It
Optional Body Functions

Hobbies and Crafts

Self-Actualization Through Macramé
Cuticle Crafts
Procrastinator's Ping-Pong
Sky Diving for Shy People
Tiddlywinks for Trying Times
How to Crack Nuts with Your Teeth
Exploring Symptoms of Terminal
    Diseases as a Hobby
Making rugs from Your Old
    Underwear
Home Decorating with Personal
    X-Rays
How to Draw Genitalia

Please return your requests as soon as possible. Applications received after 2010 will not be accepted.

©1995 Whole Person Press 210 W Michigan Duluth MN 55802   (800) 247-6789

176 NIGHT SKY

In this awe-inspiring guided image participants search the heavens for a sense of cosmic meaning and connectedness.

GOALS

To tap into creative energies and explore inner truths.

To engender a sense of connection to the cosmos.

TIME FRAME

8–10 minutes

MATERIALS NEEDED

Audio system and relaxing/energizing music (optional).

PROCESS

☞ *Make sure distractions are kept to a minium during this exercise. You may want to dim the lights and play some new age "space" music softly in the background.*

1) The trainer invites participants to indulge in an inspirational awareness-expanding exploration of a starry night.

   ➤ Settle back into your seat and gently close your eyes.

   ➤ Imagine that you are seated in a darkened Omnimax theater with a giant screen above and around you.

   ➤ Relax comfortably into the support of your plush, reclining seat.

   ➤ Take a few deep breaths to launch yourself on a cosmic adventure.

2) The trainer slowly reads the **Night Sky** script.

   ☞ *Don't hurry! Visualize the images yourself and enjoy the process as you soar through the script.*

   Occasionally people may feel anxious or uncomfortable with guided imagery. Encourage folks to trust the flow of images they experience, but remind them that they are in control of the process and can change the images at any time, or even open their eyes, if necessary, to escape an unsettling image.

   This guided image is not appropriate for individuals who are phobic or experience distortions of reality.

NIGHT SKY Script

As you relax yourself . . .
and prepare to enjoy the wide expanse of the night sky . . .
Begin to close your eyes . . . and let go . . .
Notice any part of you body . . . that feels constricted and small . . .
As you breathe . . . imagine filling that tight area with air . . .
letting it expand as you breathe in . . .
and as you breathe out . . . let this area relax . . .
Feel yourself open . . . and expand . . .
as you let go of the tension . . .

Once again . . .
allow yourself to expand as you breathe in . . .
and to relax as you breathe out . . .

Imagine that you are looking up . . . at the night sky . . .
You are outside . . . away from the lights . . .
The night is clear . . . and calm . . .
The stars are shining . . . the evening holds a quiet magic.

You notice where you are . . .
You notice the season of the year . . .

You are alone . . . but safe and calm . . . in the quiet of the night . . .
You are quiet . . . filled with a sense of awe . . .
As you gaze on the expanse of the night . . .
you notice the brilliant diamond lights . . . that blanket the heavens.

You notice a layering of the expanse . . .
stars that puncture the darkness with clarity . . .
others that dim . . .
still others only subliminal suggestions . . .
mere hints of the thousands and millions of stars not seen . . .
that extend into the infinite expanse . . . which your eyes cannot reach.

You look over the whole sky . . .
and you notice what you see . . .
as you look . . . from horizon . . . to horizon.

You focus on a cluster of stars . . .
Stars appear . . . at the edge of your vision . . .
You focus on them . . . but they disappear as you do . . .

Your eyes wander . . .
a falling star streaks across the darkness . . .

and before you get focused . . .
it disappears and vaporizes into a memory . . .
a memory that touched you . . .
a memory that you never got hold of . . .

Your eyes focus on stars that sparkle . . .
on stars that remain constant . . .
on stars that come in and out of focus . . .
seeming to disappear, then reappear at will . . .

Your eyes come to rest . . .

You focus on nothing . . .
But you take in the sense of the whole . . .
and you feel the expanse . . .
You sense the unlimited infinite . . .
without known boundaries . . . that goes on forever . . .

And you breathe . . . deeply . . .
Taking this expanse into yourself . . . fully . . .

You let go of your own boundaries . . .
you expand into the night sky . . .
you live for the moment in the wonder of the sky . . .

And you let go of your boundaries . . .
connected with awe . . . to the expanse . . .
that always holds more than you can see . . .
that seems to be bigger than your imagination . . .

And you gaze in awe . . . at the sky . . .
which goes on without ending . . . of which you are a part . . .

And allow yourself . . . to fill . . .
to expand . . . with the wonder of the moment.

When you are ready . . .
you allow yourself to return . . . from this vision.

Still open . . . unconstrained . . . relaxed . . .
having been expanded . . .
having been touched . . .
by the infinite expanse of the clear night sky . . .
that extends out forever.

This script is available on tape with background music by Steven Halpern: **Daydreams 1: Get-Aways** *(Duluth MN: Whole Person Press, 1986)*

177 PERSONAL VITALITY KIT

Everyone receives an envelope of symbolic reminders to stimulate whole person self-care.

GOALS

To reinforce self-care concepts and practices.

To encourage creativity and humor.

TIME FRAME

5 minutes (substantial preparation time for large groups)

MATERIALS NEEDED

A **Vitality Kit** for each participant.

PROCESS

☞ *In advance, prepare* **Vitality Kits** *using common small objects that can serve as metaphors for the concepts you would like to introduce or reinforce. See the list on p 128 for ideas to get your creative juices flowing. Then make up your own kit to fit you, your audience, and your subject. Put the objects in envelopes labeled* **Vitality Kit.**

1) The trainer distributes **Personal Vitality Kits** and guides participants through activities and demonstrations illustrating whole person self-care concepts, represented by each item.

2) The trainer encourages participants to use these common items regularly, as self-care cues.

VARIATIONS

■ Give kits to small groups and have them brainstorm connections to whole person self-care for each item.

■ A great opening or closing activity, this energizer could easily be expanded into a major content presentation, using the items in the **Vitality Kit** to illustrate key points. You could use each item as the focus for brief interaction exercise or demonstration (eg. your paper clip represents creativity. With a partner brainstorm 25 uses for a paper clip).

VITALITY KIT INGREDIENTS

PHYSICAL self-care
(eating, exercise, relaxation, addictions, attention to health)

rubber band (stretching, relaxation, exercise)
dry bean (healthy eating)

MENTAL self-care
(learning, creativity, problem-solving)

paper clip (creativity, organization)
thumbtack or pushpin (stay smart as a tack—think!)

EMOTIONAL self-care
(feelings, moods, coping skills)

computer label (re-label situations, acknowledge and name feelings)
balloon (take a deep breath, blow worries away, light-heartedness)

SPIRITUAL self-care
(values, faith, meaning, forgiveness, ritual)

telephone message sheet (stay in touch with your core)
kitchen match (igniting spirit, shedding light on issues)

LIFESTYLE self-care
(stress management, choices, balance, environment)

safety pin (holding life together, coping, rescue in a pinch)
penny (flip for lifestyle choices, time and energy spending patterns)

INTERPERSONAL self-care
(family, relationships)

paper reinforcement (reminder of need for contact, circle of friendship)
yarn (connectedness, telling stories)

©1995 Whole Person Press 210 W Michigan Duluth MN 55802   (800) 247-6789

178 SIGHTS FOR SORE EYES

In this revitalizing self-care break participants practice four techniques for relieving tension and strain in an often-neglected body part.

GOALS

To learn strategies for reducing eyestrain and tension.

To provide a relaxation break.

GROUP SIZE

Unlimited.

TIME FRAME

1–2 minutes each

PROCESS

1) The trainer asks participant for data about sources of eye strain and tension.

   ✔ How many of you regularly use word processors, computers or other video display terminals at work or at home?

   ✔ How many people work at jobs that require a large amount of reading?

   ✔ How many of you spend time daily in fluorescent lighting or other environments that irritate their eyes?

   ✔ How many people occasionally or regularly experience eye fatigue, tension, or strain?

2) The trainer notes that most people accumulate tension in the area of the eyes in response to these and other stressors.

3) Participants are invited to sample several techniques for relieving tension and strain in this area.

   ☞ *These four energizers can be presented all at once in sequence, or one at a time, spread out as mini-breaks during a longer session.*

A. Breathe and Blink

1) The trainer begins with the simplest treat for the eyes—a healthy dose of oxygen.

   ➤ Breathe deeply and blink your eyes several times. This technique increases blood flow and brings additional oxygen to the eyes.

   ➤ Try it again now—and several more times later in the session.

B. Warm Bath

1) The trainer notes that when your eyes get tired, your whole body feels tired. He then leads the group through a revitalizing "bath" for tired eyes, demonstrating the process as he describes it.

   ➤ Begin by rubbing your palms together until they are warm.

   ➤ Close your eyes and cover them completely with your warmed palms. Relax. Open your eyes in the darkness.

   ➤ Breathe deeply several times while cradling your head in your hands.

   ➤ Close your eyes again, and lift your head.

   ➤ Now exhale forcefully, releasing all remaining tension while you slowly open your eyes again.

C. Eyeball Calisthenics

1) The trainer reminds participants that the eye, like any other body part, benefits from deliberate exercise to strengthen muscles and reduce tension. He invites the group to join in some eyeball calisthenics that can be done several times a day.

   ➤ Close your eyes if you wish, and cup them in your palms. Relax in this position as much as possible.

   ➤ Now move your eyeballs as far to the right as possible. Then far to the left. Now up and down as far as you can stretch.

   ➤ Now roll your eyes around clockwise.

2) Before moving on, the trainer notes that for maximum benefit, each of these routines should be repeated 5–10 times in each direction.

D. Black as Night   ·

1) Participants are invited to give their eyes a well deserved "rest."

   ➤ Close your eyes and cup them in your palms.

   ➤ Visualize "black" as though you are in a dark room with your eyes open.

   ➤ Let any points of distraction dissolve into blackness.

   ➤ Relax and enjoy the vision of total darkness.

2) The trainer closes by reminding participants to try these revitalizing breaks several times a day for tension prevention and suggests that people try them as needed for headache relief.

TRAINER'S NOTES

*Submitted by Larry Tobin, from his intriguing daily wellness planner, **Time Well Spent** (Portland OR: Jade Mountain Press).*

179 STIMULATE AND INTEGRATE

This lively exercise provides motion which integrates both sides of the body while stimulating the mind.

GOALS

To become energized and mentally alert.

TIME FRAME

4–5 minutes

PROCESS

1) The trainer acknowledges that participants may need a break from mental activity and introduces the stimulating and integrating functions of cross-patterning exercises.

- **Simple movement is a health and energy break** that will rejuvenate your mind as well as your body and spirit. A few minutes of rhythmic movement can shake the cobwebs from your brain, revitalize your vision, and change your mood. Cross-patterning exercises like the one we are going to practice can release tight muscles, balance posture, integrate both sides of your body, and promote feelings of relaxation.

- **The technique of cross-patterning promotes sensory integration** by alternating movements that cross over your body's mid-line. The special education teachers and occupational therapists who use these techniques believe the rotational patterns stimulate the right and left hemispheres of the brain, integrating and awakening both the logical and creative dimensions.

2) The trainer asks participants to stand up and spread out in the room, allowing themselves an arm's length of space around them. When everyone has an area in which to move freely, she explains how to perform the cross-crawl exercise.

- ➤ Stand up with your feet slightly apart and your hands hanging loosely down at your side.

- ➤ Alternate stretching your right and left arm up above you, as if you were picking apples off a tree. Repeat ten times.

  ☞ *Encourage people to breathe deeply with each exchange.*

➤ Now alternate crossing your right hand to your left shoulder and your left hand to your right shoulder. Repeat the crossovers ten times.

➤ Now raise your left knee to meet your right hand at about waist height, then raise your right knee to meet your left hand. Repeat ten times as if running in place.

3) The trainer closes by recommending that participants experiment with these techniques several times a day to prevent mental and physical fatigue.

VARIATIONS

■ As a warm-up to further dialogue between two group members, add this variation to the routine. Group members stand facing a partner and gently slap their right hand on their partner's right hand. Then cross over to hit their left hand on their partner's left hand. Repeat ten times.

TRAINER'S NOTES

Submitted by Larry Tobin and Mary O'Brien Sippel. Chalktalk information supplied by Joyce Hidahl, OTR.

180 STRIKE THREE

This touching reading offers a childlike truth about healthy self-esteem.

GOALS

To stimulate positive self-esteem.

TIME

3 minutes

MATERIALS

Strike Three script.

PROCESS

☞ *This reading would make an excellent wrap up for the **Self-Esteem Pyramid**, p 15, or any discussion of self-esteem.*

1) The trainer introduces the reading, making whatever content bridge is appropriate.

2) The trainer reads the **Strike Three** script.

*We found this anonymous treasure in Jack Canfield and Mark Victor Hanson's memorable collection, **Chicken Soup for the Soul** (Deerfield Beach FL: Health Communications, Inc, 1993). For more information on Jack Canfield and his seminars, pleases call 1-800-2-ESTEEM.*

STRIKE THREE Script

A little boy was overheard talking to himself as he strode through his back-yard, baseball cap in place and toting ball and bat. "I'm the greatest baseball player in the world," he said proudly. Then he tossed the ball in the air, swung and missed. Undaunted, he picked up the ball, threw it into the air and said to himself, "I'm the greatest player ever!" He swung at the ball again, and again he misses. He paused a moment to examine bat and ball carefully. Then once again he threw the ball into the air and said, "I'm the greatest baseball player who ever lived." He swung the bat hard and again missed the ball.

"Wow!" he exclaimed. "What a pitcher!"

Resources

GUIDE TO THE RESOURCES SECTION

This resources section is intended to provide assistance for planning and preparation as you develop and expand your wellness training and health promotion consulting in various settings.

TIPS FOR TRAINERS p. 136

Ideas for engaging all seven modes of intelligence (verbal, logical, visual, kinesthetic, musical, intrapersonal, and interpersonal) in designing presentations, courses, and workshops.

EDITORS' CHOICE p. 139

Recommendations from the editors on their favorite exercises from **Wellness 5** and hints for on-the-job wellness training.

Four****Exercises: The Best of Wellness 5 p. 139
Especially for the Workplace p. 141

WINNING COMBINATIONS p. 143

Outlines for sessions of varying length using exercises from **Wellness 5** in combination. Plus notes on natural companion processes from other **Structured Exercises** volumes.

EAP and Health Promotion Presentations (90 min to 2 hours)
Risk Factors and Self-Care Workshop (1–2 hours)

ANNOTATED INDEXES to Wellness 5 p. 145

Guides to specific content segments and group activities incorporated in exercises from **Wellness 5**, identified by page reference, time frame, brief description, and comments on use.

Index to CHALKTALKS p. 145
Index to DEMONSTRATIONS p. 147
Index to PHYSICAL ENERGIZERS p. 148
Index to MENTAL ENERGIZERS p. 149
Index to RELAXATION ROUTINES p. 150

CONTRIBUTORS/EDITORS p. 151

Data on trainers who have shared their best process ideas in this volume. All are highly skilled educators and most provide in-house training, consultation, or workshops that may be valuable to you in planning comprehensive wellness programs. Many contributors are also established authors of well-respected materials on stress, wellness, and training issues.

WHOLE PERSON PUBLICATIONS p. 155

Descriptions of trainer-tested audio, video, and print resources available from the stress and wellness specialists.

©1995 Whole Person Press 210 W Michigan Duluth MN 55802   (800) 247-6789

TIPS FOR TRAINERS

Designing Presentations and Workshops Using
Structured Exercises in Wellness Promotion Volume 5

Wellness is a complicated issue for most of us—evaluating lifestyle habits and getting motivated to change our patterns takes our best problem-solving skills. That's why Exercise 162, **Seven Ways of Knowing** (p. 76) may be the most important process in this volume for you as a trainer. Gardner's revolutionary concept of multiple intelligences challenges us as educators to examine our teaching style to make sure we are activating all types of intelligence in our program planning and presentation.

Start by looking closely at the seven types of intelligence described on pages 78–80. You probably engage several of these modes in any presentation— telling stories or jokes *(verbal/linguistic)*, inserting a puzzle or brain teaser for effect *(logical/mathematical)*, providing visual aids with charts, diagrams, slides, etc *(visual/spatial)*, and encouraging individual reflection and application of your content presentation *(intrapersonal)*. Most trainers these days provide at least a bit of time for small group discussion or sharing with a neighbor *(interpersonal)*, but rarely do trainers feel comfortable asking audiences to role play *(kinesthetic)*, or join in a *musical/rhythmic* exercise.

Unfortunately, most of us adults rarely exercise these last two modes—having been socialized to leave these areas to the professionals. Perhaps your most potent tools as a trainer are the awareness that all seven types of intelligence are equally important and your willingness to create a learning experience where participant can access then all.

The thirty-eight exercises in this volume (as well as all others in the **Stress Management** and **Wellness Promotion** series), are designed to appeal to all seven ways of knowing. Almost all activate the *intrapersonal* dimension through individual reflection, and *interpersonal* dimension through a shared activity, group brainstorming, and/or sharing in pairs, small groups, or the large group.

Most of the longer processes, such as **Family Health Tree** , p. 15, and **Life Themes**, p. 23, typically use strategies that engage multiple intelligences. **Seven Ways of Knowing**, p. 76, is intended to explore each approach in depth. **Personal Vitality Kit**, p. 127, could easily be expanded to include multi-modal reminders of well-being. If you're trying to appeal to a certain mode of intelligence, try one of the following.

VERBAL/LINGUISTIC

145C I See Myself	p. 3	*describing personal qualities*
146 Fact or Fiction	p. 4	*reporting self-care behaviors*
148 Self-Esteem Pyramid	p. 10	*verbalizing personal strengths*

156 **Assertive Consumer**   p. 50   *complaint/commendation letters*
156 **Take the Pledge**   p. 110 *paraphrasing a familiar commitment*
175 **Ludicrous Workshops** p. 121 *writing humorous course titles*
180 **Strike Three**   p. 134 *story telling/listening*

LOGICAL/MATHEMATICAL

145A **Anchors Aweigh**   p. 1   *making analogies*
147 **Health Transcript**   p. 7   *evaluating past performance*
149 **TO DO Lists**   p. 12   *ranking priorities*
150 **Family Health Tree**   p. 15   *ordering and classifying*
152 **Pie Charts**   p. 33   *symbolic mathematical representation*
155 **Values and Self-Care** p. 45   *ranking, comparing and contrasting*
163 **Relationship Report**   p. 85   *checklist evaluation and comparison*
167 **If . . . Then**   p. 99   *cause and effect*

VISUAL/SPATIAL

150 **Family Health Tree**   p. 15   *genogram diagram*
153 **State Flag**   p. 37   *graphic representation of internal state*
157 **Mealtime Meditation**   p. 56   *visualization of hungers*
159 **Imagery: Healthy Heart** p. 62 *cardiovascular fitness visualization*
164 **Spiritual Fingerprint** p. 89   *artistic expression of inner truth*
169 **Self-Care Bouquet**   p. 106 *affirmation drawing*
176 **Night Sky**   p. 124 *awe-inspiring visualization*

BODY/KINESTHETIC

145B **Ball Toss**   p. 2   *reinforce names with movement*
159 **Imagery: Healthy Heart** p. 62 *explore circulatory system with imagery*
160 **Seventh Inning Stretch** p. 68 *memorable relaxation metaphors*
172 **Cleansing Breath**   p. 115 *focused breathing for relaxation*
173 **For the Health of It** p. 117 *reinforce exercise through dance*
178 **Sights for Sore Eyes** p. 129 *soothing through touch*
179 **Stimulate & Integrate** p. 132 *sensory integration movements*

MUSICAL/RHYTHMIC

145A **Anchors Aweigh**   p. 1   *add the sound of your boat to intros*
164 **Spiritual Fingerprint** p. 89   *type of music may influence creations*
172 **Cleansing Breath**   p. 115 *rhythmic Yoga breathing*
173 **For the Health of It** p. 117 *music evokes body movement*
174 **Healthy Singalong**   p. 119 *message in the music*
179 **Stimulate & Integrate** p. 132 *healthy rhythmic flow*

INTRAPERSONAL

148 **Self-Esteem Pyramid**   p. 10   *identify positive qualities in self*
149 **TO DO Lists**   p. 12   *explore personal goals*
151 **Life Themes**   p. 15   *discover recurring inner themes*
155 **Values and Self-Care** p. 45   *affirm motivating values*

157 **Mealtime Meditation**   p. 56   *visualization to identify inner needs*
163 **Relationship Report**   p. 85   *assess impact of others*
164 **Spiritual Fingerprint** p. 89   *get in touch with creative core*
165 **Leisure Pursuits**   p. 93   *uncover primary motivators*
169 **Self-Care Bouquet**   p. 106   *explore areas in need of support*
170 **Take the Pledge**   p. 110   *decide on resolutions for change*

INTERPERSONAL

All the Icebreakers engage participants in conversation and self-disclosure with others. Most exercises in the Wellness Explorations, Self-Care, and Planning/Closure sections involve some time in small group interaction, and these three focus primarily on interpersonal knowing:

161 **Mental Health Index**   p. 71   *group generates all the data*
166 **Commercial Success**   p. 97   *collaborative creative effort*
171 **Choose Wellness**   p. 113   *great show of group solidarity*

The principles of activating multiple intelligences are your invitation to new dimensions in training. Use this model to assess your strengths as a teacher, and then take up the creative challenge to activate all seven ways of knowing with every audience or subject matter.

To exercise your mental agility and push your boundaries a bit, take a self-care topic and use the suggestions on p. 82–83 to imagine how you might approach the issue through each mode of intelligence. For example, if your topic were *vitamins*, you could ask participants to:

Verbal/Linguistic: Create a poem or jump rope chant that extols the sources and virtues of different vitamins;

Logical/Mathematical: Classify a group of vitamins in five different ways;

Visual/Spatial: Make a diagram or poster to teach third graders (or senior citizens) about vitamins;

Body/Kinesthetic: Create appropriate, memorable gestures for each vitamin, or make up a drama with people playing the roles of different vitamins;

Musical/Rhythmic: Make up a sound and rhythm for your assigned vitamin and use it to teach others about its qualities;

Interpersonal: In small groups, discuss the pros and cons of taking vitamin supplements, then develop a resolution on vitamins to be issued by the Surgeon General;

Intrapersonal: Write a personal statement: *If I could be a vitamin, which one would I be and why?*, or keep a journal of your week with vitamins.

What we call creativity may be primarily the ability to exercise multiple intelligences and combine their power to solve problems—or present content material—in a new way. Be adventurous.

EDITORS' CHOICE

Although all 36 exercises in this volume are practical, creative, and time-tested, we must admit that we use some more often than others. When people call us and ask for suggestions about which exercises to incorporate into their workshop designs, we typically recommend some of our favorites—processes that we have worked over and over again with many audiences, readings and activities that are guaranteed to charm a group. We call these our FOUR****STAR choices.

Four****Star Exercise	Page	Comments (Timing)
146 Fact or Fiction	p. 4	This playful exercise engages folks in a stimulating search for truth about each other's health habits. Fun and adaptable for any group. (10–15 min)
150 Family Health Tree	p. 15	The genogram is one of Sandy's favorite tools for gathering and recording family history. Always a big hit with individuals and groups exploring family connections to current health and behavior issues. (50–60 min)
152 Pie Charts	p. 33	Simple, powerful metaphor for quick assessment of health care actions and attitudes. Easily adaptable to general or specific content. (20–30 min)
153 State Flag	p. 37	Highly recommended as an imaginative process for exploring personal health and well-being. (10–15 min)
156 Assertive Consumer	p. 49	Stir people to action and practice proactive wellness behaviors with this empowering letter-writing campaign. (40–50 min)
157 Mealtime Meditation	p. 56	We wrote this guided image for ourselves, and pass it on for others to enjoy as a prelude to a relaxing, healthy meal. Try it! (10–15 min)
164 Spiritual Fingerprint	p. 89	For groups willing to roll up their sleeves and delve into a creative activity, this exploration of personal spirituality is likely to be both fun and meaningful. (60 min)

166 Commercial Success p. 97 Don't be surprised if in the process of
trying to sell others on ideas of wellness,
you buy the "product" yourself. That's
the point of this dynamic closing
exercise. (15–20 min)

173 For the Health of It p. 117 There's nothing like a polka to get folks
up and moving, stimulate laughter, and
recharge a group with energy. (5–10 min)

174 Healthy Singalong p. 119 Nancy loves to get a group energized
with playful songs, and this one is sure to
engage everyone in a lively chorus of
sounds and movement. (3–5 min)

180 Strike Three p. 134 This humorous, touching reading is the
perfect accompaniment for a session on
self-esteem. (3 min)

ESPECIALLY FOR THE WORKPLACE

Most of the exercises in this volume are "generic" wellness processes that can be easily adapted to a variety of settings. When you are asked to conduct on-site health promotion programs you may want to select content or processes that are particularly applicable in the workplace. All of the exercises listed below should be appropriate in nearly any job setting.

Workplace Exercise	Page	Comments (Timing)
146 Fact or Fiction	p. 4	An intriguing process for getting to know others in your group by guessing their true health habits. (10–15 min)
149 To Do Lists	p. 12	This get-acquainted exercise includes a tool work groups will treasure: A TO DO list that makes long and short-term goal-setting a breeze. (15–20 min)
152 Pie Charts	p. 33	Extremely powerful and infinitely flexible assessment tool. Guaranteed to generate insights. (20–30 min)
154 Work APGAR	p. 44	Perfect tool for quick, easy assessments of employee satisfaction in the workplace. (10–15 min)
158 Healthy Exercise	p. 61	Ideal for worksite wellness programs and brown bag seminars. Easily adapted for shorter or longer sessions. (20–60 min)
162 Seven Ways of Knowing	p. 76	Creative, affirming exploration of seven forms of intelligence. Great for creative problem solving and team-building. (60–90 min)
165 Leisure Pursuits	p. 93	This exercise is ideal for wellness groups or anyone seeking a balance between work and leisure time. Using versatile pie charts for assessment, people discover their priorities and plan leisure activities that meet their needs. (20–30 min)
167 If...Then	p. 99	Focus on health behaviors affecting work, or adapt this exercise to any situation where you want to imagine possible outcomes of actions taken. (15–20 min)

171 Choose Wellness   p. 113   Don Ardell's wellness litany asserts
   Anyway   wellness choices we can celebrate.
                                     Read it, sing and shout it with your
                                     group, frame it and hang it in your
                                     workplace or home. (5–10 min)

175 Ludicrous   p. 121   Hilarious energizing activity guaranteed
   Workshops   to spark the creativity of any group.
                                     (15–20 min)

177 Personality   p. 127   Whole person self-care belongs in the
   Vitality Kit   workplace as well as home. Encourage
                                     creativity and humor using common
                                     office objects to symbolize self-care
                                     concepts and practices. (5 min)

178 Sights for Sore Eyes p. 129   Workers using computers or other video
                                     display terminals will welcome this
                                     refreshing series of fast, easy energizers
                                     to combat eye fatigue. (1–2 min each)

180 Strike Three   p. 134   This wonderful reading is an excellent
                                     companion piece for any session on self-
                                     esteem, confidence, or optimism. (3 min)

WINNING COMBINATIONS

EAP and Health Promotion Presentations (30–90 min)

If you are charged with promoting a wellness program or introducing EAP services in a workplace, a participatory learning experience is the most effective motivational tool available. Using the structured exercises in this volume you can spice up your marketing campaign as you get people actively involved in self-care issues. Consider using one of these approaches.

FITNESS FOCUS

When it come to getting people geared up about fitness, it's tough to beat the **Healthy Exercise** video/reflection/discussion process (Exercise 158, p. 61, 20–60 min), which features ordinary folk—rather than fitness freaks—struggling to get/stay healthy.

The sixty-minute process includes an icebreaker, personal reflection worksheets, small group sharing and a planning process, as well as a brief visualization/ relaxation routine. If healthy eating is a potential hook to capture participants, try the unusual and affirming **Mealtime Meditation** (Exercise 157, p. 56, 10– 15 min).

MENTAL HEALTH FOCUS

Motivating people to seek help with personal or family problems is no picnic, but it is possible.

Begin the session with introductions, using the format from Exercise 145C, **I See Myself** (p. 3, 5 min). Then engage people in defining mental health and recognizing common mental health problems using Exercise 161, **Mental Health Index** (p. 71, 30–45 min). As part of *Step 7*, distribute information about EAP services or upcoming wellness programs.

Since relationshop dynamics and work issues are such important components of mental well-being, try Exercise 163, **Relationship Report Card** (p. 85, 30– 40 min) and/or **Work APGAR** (Exercise 154, p. 40, 10–15 min) if you have time.

Close with the intriguing floral essences metaphor **Self-Care Bouquet** (Exercise 169, p. 106, 20–30 min).

If you have time for group energizers, introduce the **Cleansing Breath** (Exercise 172, p. 115, 3–5 min) or the **Personal Vitality Kit** (Exercise 177, p. 127, 5–10 min) to stimulate creative self-care habits.Risk Factors and Health Promotion Workshop (90 min to 2 hrs).

Risk Factors and Self-Care Workshop (90 min to 2 hrs)

If you're looking for a new approach to wellness, consider using the **Family Health Tree** (p. 15, 50–60 min) as the focal point for a workshop on personal health promotion. Most folks are intrigued by their family history, but very few have ever considered their heritage from a health perspective exclusively.

To set the tone for personal exploration of well-being, begin with Exercise 147, **Health Transcript** (p. 7, 15–20 min), which challenges participants to assess all dimensions of their health—physical, mental, spiritual, relational, emotional, leisure. This whole person base will help people tune in to the wide variety of health issues that may emerge as they draw their family medical (and psycho-social) history.

> Since most families will reveal history of heart disease, you may want to include Exercise 159, **Imagery for a Healthy Heart** (p. 63, 10–15 min) as a skill-building component of your presentation/workshop. Nearly everyone would benefit from a daily dosage of this powerful, preventive, healing visualization.

Close the session with a reminder about the impact of our day to day behavior choices as they interact with our genetic and environmental heritage. Use the worksheet and open-ended format of Exercise 167, **If . . . Then** (p. 99, 15–20 min) once to help people project negative consequences of their health history and current health patterns. Then distribute a second worksheet and challenge people to imagine more positive health outcomes—and strategies they might use to reach them.

As a last hurrah, join in a group affirmation of the wellness lifestyle, using Exercise 171, **Choose Wellness Anyway** (p. 113, 5–10 min).

If you're adventurous, lead the group in a rousing chorus of *If You're Healthy and You Know It,* Exercise 174 (p. 119, 3–5 min) as an icebreaker, or after the Health Transcripts.

ANNOTATED INDEXES

Index to CHALKTALKS

152 Pie Charts   p. 33 Whole person self-care.

150 Family Health Tree   p. 16 Personal health is often a family legacy
                                     of both strengths and weakness.
                              p. 16 Definition and purpose of genogram
                              p. 20 Tips for exploring family history.

151 Life Themes   p. 23 Positive and negative life themes can be
                                     altered with perceptiveness, planning,
                                     and practice.
                              p. 28 What is a ritual and how can it be used to
                                     promote healthy life themes?
                              p. 30 How to use the three P's—
                                     perceptiveness, planning, and practice.

154 Work Apgar   p. 40 History and purpose of APGAR scale.
                              p. 42 Worksite wellness is important.

155 Values and   p. 45 Values shape self-care choices.
Self-Care Choices   Problems develop when values are
                                     unclear or conflicted.

156 Assertive Consumer   p. 50 Characteristics of assertive consumers.
                              p. 52 Guidelines for assertive communication.
                              p. 54 Risks and benefits of assertive behavior.

157 Mealtime Meditation   p. 56 Mealtime is an opportunity for self-care.

159 Imagery for a   p. 63 Guided imagery can enhance health
Healthy Heart   and healing.

161 Mental Health Index   p. 72 Six mental health problems:
                                     adjustment problems, anxiety/panic,
                                     post-traumatic stress disorder, family
                                     problems, alcohol, drugs and gambling
                                     addictions, and depression.
                              p. 74 Guidelines for when and how to seek
                                     professional help.

162 Seven Ways of   p. 77 The complex nature of intelligence.
Knowing   p. 78 Concept of multiple intelligences and the
                                     seven ways of knowing.
                              p. 82 Strategies for enhancing seven types of
                                     intelligence.

163 Relationship   p. 85 Healthy relationships.
    Report Card   p. 87 Tips for developing healthy relationships.

164 Spiritual Fingerprint p. 90 What is spirituality?
                             p. 92 Care for your spirit.

169 Self-Care Bouquet   p. 106 Bach flower remedies for harmony and
                                     balance.

172 Cleansing Breath   p. 115 Breathing and Yoga.

173 For the Health of It p. 117 Health benefits of dancing.

179 Stimulate and   p. 132 Cross-patterning exercise for sensory
    Integrate   integration.

©1995 Whole Person Press 210 W Michigan Duluth MN 55802   (800) 247-6789

Index to DEMONSTRATIONS

150 Family Health Tree   p. 17 Demonstrates how to understand a
                                    genogram and use it as a tool for
                                    exploring family history. (30–50 min)

162 Seven Ways of   p. 77 On the spot IQ test demonstrates
    Knowing   seven intelligent approaches to problem
                                    solving. (3–5 min)

172 Cleansing Breath   p. 115 Demonstration of the basic Yoga
                                    alternate side breathing technique.
                                    (3–5 min)

173 For the Health of It p. 118 Lively dance steps are taught by the
                                    trainer and enjoyed by participants.
                                    (5–10 min)

178 Sights for   p. 130 Trainer shows participants how to treat
    Sore Eyes   themselves to a revitalizing "bath" for
                                    tired eyes. (1–2 min)

179 Stimulate and   p. 132 Step-by-step instructions for do-it-
    Integrate   yourself sensory integration. (4–5 min)

Index to PHYSICAL ENERGIZERS

145 Ball Toss   p. 2   An imaginary game of catch helps people get acquainted. (2–3 min)

166 Commercial Success   p. 97   Participants create and perform a dynamic commercial to sell wellness concepts to the public. (10–12 min)

173 For the Health of It   p. 117   Participants get energized as they kick up their heels. (5–10 min)

174 Healthy Singalong   p. 119   This lively song involves clapping, running-in-place, and laughing. (3–5 min)

179 Stimulate and Integrate   p. 132   Cross-patterning movement stimulates the body and mind. (4–5 min)

Index to MENTAL ENERGIZERS

162 Seven Ways of   p. 76   Seven forms of intelligence are explored
Knowing in this fascinating exercise. Easily
modified for shorter times. (60–90 min)

164 Spiritual Fingerprint p. 89   Playful, right-brain process of creating an
art form to represent personal spirituality.
(90 min)

166 Commercial   p. 97   Synthesize learning by creating and
Success performing a commercial to sell key ideas
to the group. (15–20 min)

171 Choose Wellness   p. 113   Principles of wellness are asserted in this
Anyway high-spirited litany. (5–10 min)

174 Healthy Singalong   p. 119   This playful, song provides heatlhy
remedies in a refreshing, light-hearted
break. (3–5 min)

175 Ludicrous   p. 121   Hilarious exercise to tickle funny bones
Workshops and refresh weary minds. (15-20 min)

177 Personal   p. 127   Participants are challenged to transform
Vitality Kit a packet of common, everyday objects
into tools for self-care. (5 min)

180 Strike Three   p. 134   Delightful story depicting healthy self-
esteem and unwavering optimism.
(3–5 min)

Index to RELAXATION ROUTINES

157 Mealtime Meditation p. 56 Participants relax and tune in to the natural rhythms of their body in this calming visualization. Ideal for longer workshops with a lunch break. (10–15 min)

158 Healthy Exercise p. 61 The three-minute relaxation sequence at the end of the **Healthy Choices** video provides motivation for healthy exercise. (3 min)

159 Imagery for a Healthy Heart p. 63 Participants use powerful sensory imaging techniques to visualize healthy circulation and affirm their capacity for healing and renewal. (10–15 min)

172 Cleansing Breath p. 115 This Yoga breathing technique is a powerful natural tranquilizer. Easy to learn and do, any time, any place. (3–5 min)

176 Night Sky p. 124 An awe-inspiring guided image that explores the wonder of the universe and our connections to it. (8–10 min)

178 Sights for Sore Eyes p. 129 Relief for tired eyes comes with these four soothing techniques to rest and revitalize. Can be put to immediate use at home or at the office. (1–2 min each)

CONTRIBUTORS

Donald B Ardell, Director, Wellness Institute, University of Central Florida. Orlando FL 32816. 407/823-2453. Don is the author of the landmark book **High Level Wellness: An Alternative to Doctors, Drugs, and Disease** and ten other books, including **Die Healthy** and **Freedom, Self-Management, and the Wellness Orgasm** (with Grant Donovan). He also publishes the quarterly **Ardell Wellness Report**, of which there are now 33 editions in print (for a sample copy send a SASE to Dr Ardell).

Lyman Coleman, MDiv, PhD. Serendipity House, Box 1012, Littleton CO 80160. 303/798-1313. Founder and director of Serendipity Workshops, Lyman has spent the past 30 years training over 150,000 church leaders of all denominations in small group processes. Author of scores of books, including a small group discussion version of the Bible, Lyman's innovative approach combines Bible study, group building and values orientation with personal story telling.

David G Danskin, PhD. 180 Gray Mountain Drive, Sedona AZ 86336. 602/282-2372. David, a professor emeritus of Kansas State University, is the author of **Quicki-Mini Stress-Management Strategies for Work, Home, Leisure** and is co-author with Dorothy V. Danskin of **Quicki-Mini Stress-Management Strategies for You, a Disabled Person**. He is also senior author of **Biofeedback: an Introduction and Guide**. David is now enjoying his retirement in Arizona.

Lois B Hart, President, Leadership Dynamics. 10951 Isabelle Road, Lafayette CO 80026-9209. 303/666-4046. Author of several excellent training manuals including **Connections: 125 Activities for Successful Workshops**, **Faultless Facilitation: A Resource Guide and Instruction Manual**, **50 Activities to Develop Leaders**, **Training Methods That Work**, and **Learning from Conflict: A Conference and Workshop Planner's Manual**, Lois offers workshops, consultation, and presentations to all kinds of organizations who are interested in the development of their leaders and employees.

Krysta Eryn Kavenaugh, MA, CSP. 955 Lake Drive, St. Paul MN 55120. 800/829-8437 (w) 612/725-6763 (h). Krysta is a speaker, trainer, and consultant. Her mission is to take people "into the heart of wisdom." She speaks with style, substance, and spirit. She is also the managing editor of **Marriage** magazine. Her favorite keynote topic is "Romancing Yourself: Taking Care of You is Taking Care of Business." She also speaks on proactive support teams, turning adversity to our advantage, ecology, and customized business topics.

Julie Lusk, MEd. Lewis-Gale Clinic, 1802 Braeburn Drive, Salem VA 24153. 703/772-3736. Julie is the editor of **30 Scripts for Relaxation, Imagery, and Inner Healing** (volumes 1 and 2). She works as the director of the Health Management Center at Lewis-Gale Clinic and is the founder of the Alive and Well Coalition in Roanoke VA. She leads workshops worldwide on a variety of topics and develops wellness programs for businesses, colleges, and communities. Julie is a licensed professional counselor and has taught Yoga since 1977.

Belleruth Naparstek, MA. 2460 Fairmount Blvd, Suite 320, Cleveland Heights OH, 44106. 216/791-0909. Author of **Staying Well with Guided Imagery**, Belleruth was trained as a clinical social worker at the University of Chicago, and has been a practicing psychotherapist for the past thirty years. She is the creator of the **Health Journeys** audiotape series which grew out of her research and clinical practice with individuals who have life-threatening and debilitating diseases.

Price Pritchett, PhD. 13155 Noel Ct, Suite 1600, Dallas TX 75240. 214/789–7971. Price is the CEO of Pritchett & Associates Inc, a Dallas-based consulting firm specializing in organizational change. He has authored eleven books on individual and organizational effectiveness, including **You²: A High Velocity Formula for Multiplying Your Personal Effectiveness in Quantum Leaps, New Work Habits for a Radically Changing World**, and **The Employee's Survival Guide to the Stress of Organizational Change**.

Sandy Queen, Director, LIFEWORKS. PO Box 2668, Columbia MD 21045. 301/796-5310. Sandy is the founder and director of Lifeworks Inc, a training/counseling firm that specializes in helping people take a better look at their lives through humor, laughter, and play. She has developed many innovative programs in the areas of stress-reduction, humor, children's wellness, and self-esteem.

John Sippola, M.Div. 219 N 6th Ave East, Duluth MN 55805. 218-722-3381 (w). After fifteen years as director of Chaplaincy at Miller Dwan Hospital, John is currently tackling the challenges of whole person wellness in parish ministry. An innovative group leader and gifted teacher, John has specialized in mental health, drug and alcohol treatment programs, and recovery/relapse issues.

Mary O'Brien Sippel, RN, MS. Licensed Psychologist, 22 East St. Andrews, Duluth MN 55803. 218/723-6130 (w) 218/724-5935 (h). Mary has spent over twenty-five years working the field of community health and education. Her experience in teaching stress management, burnout prevention, and wellness promotion across the country has enabled her to be her own best caretaker as career woman, wife, and mother of two teenagers. Mary is currently a personal counselor and adjunct faculty member at the College of St. Scholastica, Duluth MN. She has ten publications to her credit, never tiring of sharing her enthusiasm for life both on paper and in front of her audiences.

Gabriel Smilkstein, MD. Professor, University of California–Davis Department of Family Practice, Davis CA 95616. 916/759–2370 (w). Gabe has a long-standing interest in the family and the biopsychological model of health. Author of ten textbook chapters in family medicine and over fifty papers in peer review journals, his most recent studies relating to the influence of psychosocial risk factors on pregnancy outcome indicate the importance of social support.

Sally Strosahl, MA. Marriage & Family Therapist, 116 S Westlawn, Aurora IL 60506. 708/897-9796. Sally has an MA in clinical psychology; trained at the Wholistic Health Center; researched the relationship between stress and illness. In addition to her private practice in marriage and family therapy, Sally frequently presents workshops in the areas of stress and wellness management, burnout prevention, body image and size acceptance, and marriage enrichment. She particularly enjoys working with "systems" (family, work groups, agencies, business, churches) to help enhance each member's growth and well-being.

David X Swenson, PhD. Assoc Professor of Management, College of St Scholastica, 1200 Kenwood Ave, Duluth MN 55811. 218/723-6476 (w) 218/525-3723 (h). A licensed consulting psychologist, Dave maintains a private practice in addition to his educational and therapeutic roles at the college. He provides consultation and training to human services, health, and law enforcement agencies and is the author of **Stress Managment in the Criminal Justice System**. Dave also develops stress management software.

Larry Tobin, MA. Jade Mist Press, 2529 SE 64th, Portland OR 97026. Larry is a special educator, school psychologist, and national trainer on working with troubled children. He has authored **What Do You Do with a Child Like This?**, **62 Ways to Create Change in the Lives of Troubled Children**, and **Time Well Spent**, a year-long stress management planner.

Mark Warner, EdD. Associate Professor of Health Sciences, James Madison University, Harrisonburg VA 22807. 703/568-3685. In addition to his teaching duties, Mark consults, writes, and presents on the topics of wellness promotion, leadership development, and organizational development.

FUTURE CONTRIBUTORS

If you have developed an exciting, effective exercise you'd like to share with other trainers in the field of stress or wellness, please send it to us for consideration, using the following guidelines:

- Your entry should be written in a format similiar to those in this volume.

- Contributors must either guarantee that the materials they submit are not previously copyrighted or provide a copyright release for inclusion in the Whole Person **Structured Exercises** series.

- When you have adapted the work of others, please acknowledge the original source of ideas or activities.

EDITORS

All exercises in this volume not specifically attributed to other contributors are the creative efforts of the editors, who have been designing, collecting, and experimenting with structured processes in their teaching, training, and consultation work since the late 1960s.

Nancy Loving Tubesing, EdD, holds a masters degree in group counseling and a doctorate in counselor education. Faculty Associate and Product Development Director at Whole Person Associates, Nancy is co-author of two self-help books on whole person wellness, **The Caring Question** (Minneapolis: Augsburg, 1983) and **Seeking Your Healthy Balance** (Duluth: Whole Person Press, 1991) and a score of unusual relaxation audiotapes.

Nancy also collaborated with Don Tubesing in developing creative stress management programs and packages for client groups such as the national YMCA (8-session course, **The Y's Way to Stress Management**) and Aid Association for Lutherans (The Stress Kit multimedia resource for families).

Their most recent efforts have been directed toward combining the process-oriented approach of the **Structured Exercises** series with the power of video. The resulting three six-session interactive video courses, **WellAware**, **Manage It!**, and **Managing Job Stress**, include participant booklets with worksheets that stimulate personal reflection and application of principles to specific situations, as well as a step-by-step leader manual for guiding group interaction.

Sandy Stewart Christian, MSW, is a licensed independent clinical social worker and a licensed marriage and family therapist. Prior to joining the Product Development Team at Whole Person Associates in 1994, Sandy worked for nearly seventeen years as a therapist and clinical supervisor at a private counseling agency. She was on the behavioral science faculty at the Duluth Family Practice Center for over ten years and is an adjunct faculty member at the St. Mary's Hospital Chaplaincy program in Duluth, Minnesota. In her work as a therapist, teacher, trainer, and consultant, Sandy has maintained a lively whole person focus in health and stress management.

WORKSHOPS-IN-A-BOOK

The easy-to-understand, user-friendly format of Whole Person Workshops-in-a-Book are perfect for use as:
- a classroom text, discussion guide, or participant workbook;
- a professional resource for both novice and experienced trainers;
- a personal journey for individuals.

KICKING YOUR STRESS HABITS:
A Do-it-yourself Guide for Coping with Stress
Donald A. Tubesing, PhD

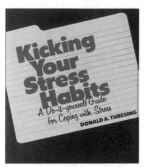

Over a quarter of a million people have found ways to deal with their everyday stress by using **Kicking Your Stress Habits**. This workshop-in-a-book actively involves the reader in assessing stressful patterns and developing more effective coping strategies with helpful "Stop and Reflect" sections in each chapter.

The 10-step planning process and 20 skills for managing stress make **Kicking Your Stress Habits** an ideal text for stress management classes in many different settings, from hospitals to universities.

Kicking Your Stress Habits / $14.95

SEEKING YOUR HEALTHY BALANCE:
A Do-it-yourself Guide to Whole Person Well-Being
Donald A. Tubesing, PhD and Nancy Loving Tubesing, EdD

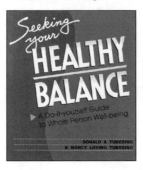

Where can people find the time and energy to "do it all" without sacrificing health and well-being? **Seeking Your Healthy Balance** helps readers discover how to develop a more balanced lifestyle by learning effective ways to juggle work, self, and others; by clarifying self-care options; and by discovering and setting personal priorities.

Seeking Your Healthy Balance asks the questions that help readers find their own answers as they pursue the path to wellness.

Seeking Your Healthy Balance / $14.95

To order, call toll free   (800) 247-6789

©1995 Whole Person Press 210 W Michigan Duluth MN 55802   (800) 247-6789

STRUCTURED EXERCISES
IN STRESS MANAGEMENT—VOLUMES 1–5

Nancy Loving Tubesing, EdD, Donald A. Tubesing, PhD,
and Sandy Stewart Christian, MSW, Editors

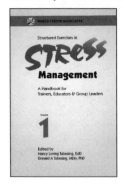

Each book in this five-volume series contains 36 ready-to-use teaching modules that involve the participant—as a whole person—in learning how to manage stress more effectively.

Each exercise is carefully designed by top stress-management professionals. Instructions are clearly written and field-tested so that even beginning trainers can smoothly lead a group through warm-up and closure, reflection and planning, action and interaction—all with minimum preparation time.

Each **Stress Handbook** is brimming with practical ideas that you can weave into your own teaching designs or mix and match to develop new programs for varied settings, audiences, and time frames. In each volume you'll find **Icebreakers, Stress Assessments, Management Strategies, Skill Builders, Action Planners, Closing Processes,** and **Group Energizers**—all with a special focus on stress management.

Stress 8 1/2" x 11" Loose-Leaf Edition—Volumes 1–5 / $54.95 per volume
Includes Worksheet Masters (see below).
Stress 6" x 9" Softcover Edition—Volumes 1–5 / $29.95 per volume

STRUCTURED EXERCISES WORKSHEET MASTERS

The Worksheet Masters for the stress and wellness **Structured Exercises** series offer full-size (8 1/2" x 11") photocopy masters. All of the worksheets and handouts for each volume are reproduced in easy-to-read print with professional graphics. All you need to do to complete your workshop preparation is run them through a copier.

Worksheet Masters are automatically included with the Loose-Leaf Editions.

Structured Exercises in Stress Management Volumes 1–5
Worksheet Masters / $9.95 per volume

Structured Exercises in Wellness Promotion Volumes 1–5
Worksheet Masters / $9.95 per volume

To order, call toll free   (800) 247-6789

©1995 Whole Person Press 210 W Michigan Duluth MN 55802   (800) 247-6789

STRUCTURED EXERCISES
IN WELLNESS PROMOTION—VOLUMES 1–5

Nancy Loving Tubesing, EdD, Donald A. Tubesing, PhD,
and Sandy Stewart Christian, MSW, Editors

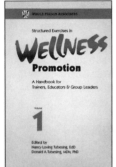

Discover the **Wellness Handbooks**—from the wellness pioneers at Whole Person Associates. Each volume in this innovative series includes 36 experiential learning activities that focus on whole person health—body, mind, spirit, emotions, relationships, and lifestyle.

The exercises, developed by an interdisciplinary pool of leaders in the wellness movement nationwide, actively encourage people to adopt wellness-oriented attitudes and to develop more responsible self-care patterns.

All process designs in the Wellness Handbooks are clearly explained and have been thoroughly field-tested with diverse audiences so that trainers can use them with confidence. **Icebreakers, Wellness Explorations, Self-Care Strategies, Action Planners, Closings,** and **Group Energizers** are all ready-to-go—including reproducible worksheets, scripts, and chalktalk outlines—for the busy professional who wants to develop unique wellness programs without spending hours in preparation.

Wellness 8 1/2" x 11" Loose-Leaf Edition—Volumes 1–5 / $54.95 per volume
Includes Worksheet Masters (see p. 154)
Wellness 6" x 9" Softcover Edition—Volumes 1–5 / $29.95 per volume

STRESS AND WELLNESS REFERENCE GUIDE
A Comprehensive Index to the Chalktalks, Processes, and Activites in the Whole Person Structured Exercises Series
Nancy Loving Tubesing, EdD

This handy index is your key to over 360 teaching designs of the ten volumes of the **Stress and Wellness Handbook** series—organized by theme, time frame, level of self-disclosure, trainer experience level, and goals. The book includes the *Tips for Trainers* sections for all ten books, with workshop outlines and suggested processes especially for the workplace—as well as annotated listings of all chalktalks, demonstrations, physical and mental energizers, relaxation techniques, and the editors' choice of favorite exercises.

The **Index** makes it easy to plan a workshop by mixing and matching exercises suitable to your audience. You'll find easy-to-read charts with a quick view of goals, times, group processes and activities—so you can find your favorites to use with any group.

Stress and Wellness Reference Guide / $29.95

©1995 Whole Person Press 210 W Michigan Duluth MN 55802   (800) 247-6789

ADDITIONAL GROUP PROCESS RESOURCES

Our group process exercises are designed to address the whole person—physical, emotional, mental, spiritual, and social. Developed for trainers by trainers, all of these topical group process resources are ready-to-use. Novice trainers will find everything they need to get started, and the expert trainer will discover new ideas and concepts to add to existing programs.

All of the exercises encourage interaction between the leader and the participants, as well as among the participants. Each exercise includes everything you need to present a meaningful program: goals, optimal group size, time frame, materials list, and complete process instructions.

PLAYFUL ACTIVITIES FOR POWERFUL PRESENTATIONS
Bruce Williamson

This book contains 40 fun exercises designed to fit any group or topic. These exercises will help you:

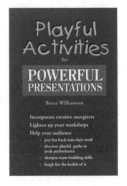

- build teamwork
- encourage laughter and playfulness
- relieve stress and tension
- free up the imagination of participants

Playful Activities for Powerful Presentations $19.95

WORKING WITH GROUPS FROM DYSFUNCTIONAL FAMILIES
Cheryl Hetherington

This collection of 29 proven group activities is designed to heal the pain that results from living in a dysfunctional family. With these exercises you can:

- promote healing • build self-esteem
- encourage sharing
- help participants acknowledge their feelings.

Working with Groups from Dysfunctional Families / $24.95

WORKSHEET MASTERS
A complete package of (8 1/2" x 11") photocopy masters is available for **Working with Groups from Dysfunctional Families**. Use the masters to conveniently duplicate handouts for each participant.

Working with Groups from Dysfunctional Families Worksheet Masters / $9.95

WORKING WITH WOMEN'S GROUPS VOLUMES 1 & 2
Louise Yolton Eberhardt

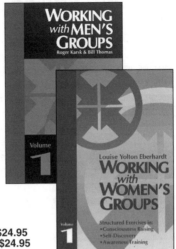

The two volumes of **Working with Women's Groups** have been completely revised and updated. These exercises will help women explore issues that are of perennial concern as well as today's hot topics.

- consciousness-raising (volume 1)
- self-discovery (volume 1)
- assertiveness training (volume 1)
- sexuality issues (volume 2)
- women of color (volume 2)
- leadership skills training (volume 2)

Working with Women's Groups Volume 1 / $24.95
Working with Women's Groups Volume 2 / $24.95

WORKING WITH MEN'S GROUPS
Roger Karsk and Bill Thomas

Also revised and updated, this volume is a valuable resource for anyone working with men's groups. The exercises cover a variety of topics, including:

- self discovery • parenting • conflict • intimacy

Working with Men's Groups / $24.95

WELLNESS ACTIVITIES FOR YOUTH VOLUMES 1 & 2
Sandy Queen

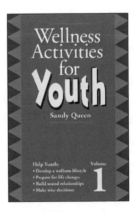

Each volume of **Wellness Activities for Youth** help leaders touch children and teenagers about wellness with an emphasis on FUN. The concepts include:

- values • stress and coping • self-esteem
- personal well-being

Wellness Activities for Youth Volume 1 / $24.95
Wellness Activities for Youth Volume 2 / $24.95

WORKSHEET MASTERS
Complete packages of full-size (8 1/2" x 11") photocopy masters that include all worksheets and handouts are available to you. Use the masters for easy duplication of the handouts for each participant.

Working with Women's Groups V. 1 & 2 Worksheet Masters / $9.95 each volume
Working with Men's Groups Worksheet Masters / $9.95
Wellness Activities for Youth V. 1 & 2 Worksheet Masters / $9.95 each volume

WORKING WITH GROUPS IN THE WORKPLACE

CONFRONTING SEXUAL HARASSMENT
Louise Yolten Eberhardt

Preventing sexual harassment requires more than just enforcing the laws—changing attitudes is just as crucial. **Confronting Sexual Harassment** contains a wealth of exercises that trainers can safely use with groups to constructively explore the issue, look at the underlying causes, understand the law, motivate men to become allies, and empower women to speak up. It's a valuable tool for private employers, government agencies, schools, religious institutions, and nonprofit organizations.

Confronting Sexual Harassment / $24.95

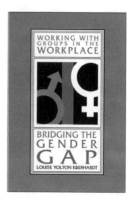

BRIDGING THE GENDER GAP
Louise Yolten Eberhardt

Bridging the Gender Gap contains 37 exercises for the trainer to use in team building, gender role awareness groups, diversity training, couples workshops, college classes, or youth seminars. The exercises encourage participants to examine gender stereotypes and attitudes, discover the effects of these attitudes, and form a shared consciousness for both genders so they can humanize their roles, relationships, and personal lives.

Bridging the Gender Gap / $24.95

To order, call toll free   (800) 247-6789

©1995 Whole Person Press 210 W Michigan Duluth MN 55802   (800) 247-6789

CELEBRATING DIVERSITY
Cheryl Hetherington

Celebrating Diversity helps people confront and question the beliefs, prejudices, and fears that can separate them from others. The 28 exercises provide valuable assistance to trainers leading groups in evaluating past experiences, exploring negative feelings, and beginning a journey toward truly celebrating the differences that unite us.

Celebrating Diversity / $24.95

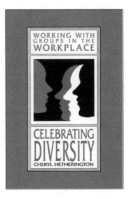

WORKING WITH GROUPS ON SPIRITUAL THEMES
Structured Exercises in Healing
Elaine Hopkins, Zo Woods, Russell Kelly,
Katrina Bentley, James Murphy

Whether spirituality is the focus of your group or is one of many issues being explored, you will find creative ideas in **Working with Groups on Spiritual Themes** that will help you initiate discussion and promote healing and personal growth. The 39 exercise are particularly effective with groups who want to explore the meaning and purpose of life. Use this book for:

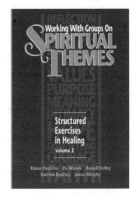

• personal growth groups • hospitals
• retreat centers • mental health facilities
• church groups • nursing homes

Spiritual Themes / $24.95

WORKSHEET MASTERS
A complete package of full-size (8 1/2" x 11") photocopy masters that includes all the worksheets and the key handouts from **Working with Groups** is available to you. Use the masters for easy duplication of the worksheets for each participant.

Confronting Sexual Harassment Worksheets / $9.95
Bridging the Gender Gap Worksheets / $9.95
Celebrating Diversity Worksheets / $9.95
Spiritual Themes Worksheets / $9.95

RELAXATION AUDIOTAPES

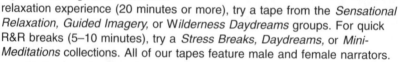

Perhaps you're an old hand at relaxation, looking for new ideas. Or maybe you're a beginner, just testing the waters. Whatever your relaxation needs, Whole Person audiotapes provide a whole family of options for reducing physical and mental stress.

Techniques range from simple breathing and stretching exercises to classic autogenic and progressive relaxation sequences, guided meditations, and whimsical daydreams. All are carefully crafted to promote whole person relaxation—body, mind, and spirit.

If you're looking for an extended relaxation experience (20 minutes or more), try a tape from the *Sensational Relaxation, Guided Imagery,* or W*ilderness Daydreams* groups. For quick R&R breaks (5–10 minutes), try a *Stress Breaks, Daydreams,* or *Mini-Meditations* collections. All of our tapes feature male and female narrators.

Audiotapes are available for $11.95 each.
Call for generous quantity discounts.

SENSATIONAL RELAXATION—$11.95 each
When stress piles up, it becomes a heavy load both physically and emotionally. These full-length relaxation experiences will teach you techniques that can be used whenever you feel that stress is getting out of control. Choose one you like and repeat it daily until it becomes second nature, then recall that technique whenever you need it—or try a new one every day.

> **Countdown to Relaxation /** Countdown 19:00, Staircase 19:00
> **Daybreak / Sundown /** Daybreak 22:00, Sundown 22:00
> **Take a Deep Breath /** Breathing for Relaxation 17:00, Magic Ball 17:00
> **Relax . . . Let Go . . . Relax /** Revitalization 27:00, Relaxation 28:00
> **StressRelease /** Quick Tension Relievers 22:00, Progressive Relaxation 20:00
> **Warm and Heavy /** Warm 24:00, Heavy 23:00

STRESS BREAKS—$11.95 each
Do you need a short energy booster or a quick stress reliever? If you don't know what type of relaxation you like, or if you are new to guided relaxation techniques, try one of our *Stress Breaks* for a quick refocusing or change of pace any time of the day.

> **BreakTime /** Solar Power 8:00, Belly Breathing 9:00, Fortune Cookie 9:00,
>   Mother Earth 11:00, Big Yawn 5:00, Affirmation 11:00
> **Natural Tranquilizers /** Clear the Deck 10:00, Body Scan 10:00,
>   99 Countdown 10:00, Calm Down 9:00, Soothing Colors 11:00,
>   Breathe Ten 9:00
> **Effortless Relaxation /** Sensory Relaxation 16:00, Breathe Away Tension 8:00,
>   Anchoring 8:00, Breathing Meditation 7:00, Pulling Strings 4:00,
>   Groans and Moans 5:00

©1995 Whole Person Press 210 W Michigan Duluth MN 55802   (800) 247-6789

DAYDREAMS—$11.95 each

Escape from the stress around you with guided tours to beautiful places. The quick escapes in our *Daydreams* tapes will lead your imagination away from your everyday cares so you can resume your tasks relaxed and comforted.

> **Daydreams 1: Getaways /** Cabin Retreat 11:00, Night Sky 10:00, Hot Spring 7:00, Mountain View 8:00, Superior Sail 8:00
>
> **Daydreams 2: Peaceful Places /** Ocean Tides 11:00, City Park 10:00, Hammock 8:00, Meadow 11:00
>
> **Daydreams 3: Relaxing Retreats /** Melting Candle 5:00, Tropical Paradise 10:00, Sanctuary 7:00, Floating Clouds 5:00, Seasons 9:00, Beach Tides 9:00

GUIDED MEDITATION—$11.95 each

Take a step beyond relaxation. The imagery in our full-length meditations will help you discover your strengths, find healing, make positive life changes, and recognize your inner wisdom.

> **Inner Healing /** Inner Healing 20:00, Peace with Pain 20:00
>
> **Personal Empowering /** My Gifts 22:00, Hidden Strengths 21:00
>
> **Healthy Balancing /** Inner Harmony 20:00, Regaining Equilibrium 20:00
>
> **Spiritual Centering /** Spiritual Centering 20:00 (male and female narration)

WILDERNESS DAYDREAMS—$11.95 each

Discover the healing power of nature with the four tapes in our *Wilderness Daydreams* series. These eight special journeys will transport you from your harried, stressful surroundings to the peaceful serenity of words and water.

> **Canoe / Rain /** Canoe 19:00, Rain 22:00
>
> **Island / Spring /** Island 19:00, Spring 19:00
>
> **Campfire / Stream /** Campfire 17:00, Stream 19:00
>
> **Sailboat / Pond /** Sailboat 25:00, Pond 25:00

MINI-MEDITATIONS—$11.95 each

These brief guided visualizations begin by focusing your breathing and uncluttering your mind, so that you can concentrate on a sequence of sensory images that promote relaxation, centering, healing, growth, and spiritual awareness.

> **Healing Visions /** Rocking Chair 5:00, Pine Forest 8:00, Long Lost Confidant 10:00, Caterpillar to Butterfly 7:00, Superpowers 9:00, Tornado 8:00
>
> **Refreshing Journeys /** 1 to 10 10:00, Thoughts Library 11:00, Visualizing Change 6:00, Magic Carpet 9:00, Pond of Love 9:00, Cruise 9:00
>
> **Healthy Choices /** Lifestyle 6:00, Eating 5:00, Exercise 3:00, Stress 5:00, Relationships 6:00, Change 7:00

MUSIC ONLY—$11.95 each

No relaxation program would be complete without relaxing melodies that can be played as background to a prepared script or that can be enjoyed as you practice a technique you have already learned. Steven Eckels composed his melodies specifically for relaxation. These "musical prayers for healing" will calm your body, mind, and spirit.

> **Tranquility /** Awakening 20:00, Repose 20:00
>
> **Harmony /** Waves of Light 30:00, Rising Mist 10:00, Frankincense 10:00, Angelica 10:00
>
> **Serenity /** Radiance 20:00, Quiessence 10:00, Evanesence 10:00

©1995 Whole Person Press 210 W Michigan Duluth MN 55802   (800) 247-6789

RELAXATION RESOURCES

Many trainers and workshop leaders have discovered the benefits of relaxation and visualization in healing the body, mind, and spirit.

30 SCRIPTS FOR RELAXATION, IMAGERY, AND INNER HEALING
Julie Lusk

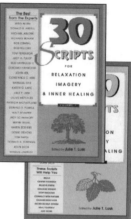

The relaxation scripts, creative visualizations, and guided meditations in these volumes were created by experts in the field of guided imagery. Julie Lusk collected their best and most effective scripts to help novices get started and experienced leaders expand their repertoire. Both volumes include information on how to use the scripts, suggestions for tailoring them to specific needs and audiences, and information on how to successfully incorporate guided imagery into existing programs.
30 Scripts / Volume 1 & 2 / $19.95 each

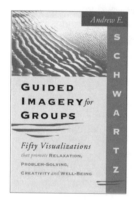

GUIDED IMAGERY FOR GROUPS
Andrew Schwartz

Ideal for courses, workshops, team building, and personal stress management, this comprehensive resource includes scripts for 50 thematic visualizations that promote calming, centering, creativity, congruence, clarity, coping, and connectedness. Detailed instructions for using relaxation techniques and guided images in group settings allow educators at all levels, in any setting, to help people tap into the healing and creative powers of imagery.
Guided Imagery for Groups / $24.95

INQUIRE WITHIN
Andrew Schwartz

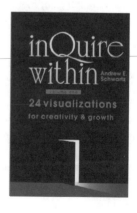

Use visualization to help people make positive changes in their life. The 24 visualization experiences in **Inquire Within** will help participants enhance their creativity, heal inner pain, learn to relax, and deal with conflict. Each visualization includes questions at the end of the process that encourage deeper reflection and a better understanding of the exercise and the response it evokes.
Inquire Within / $19.95

©1995 Whole Person Press 210 W Michigan Duluth MN 55802   (800) 247-6789